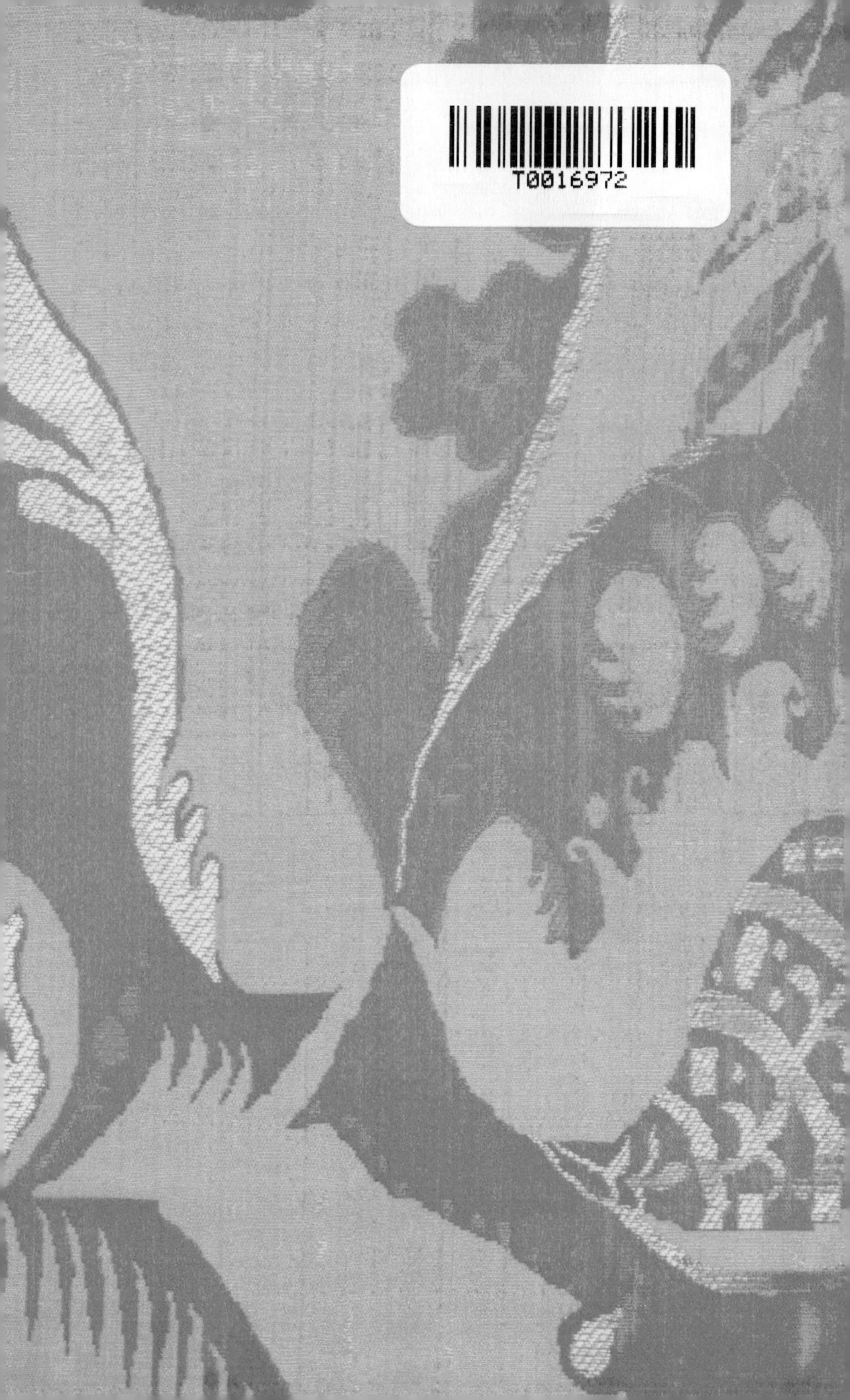

SWAMI
VIVEKANANDA

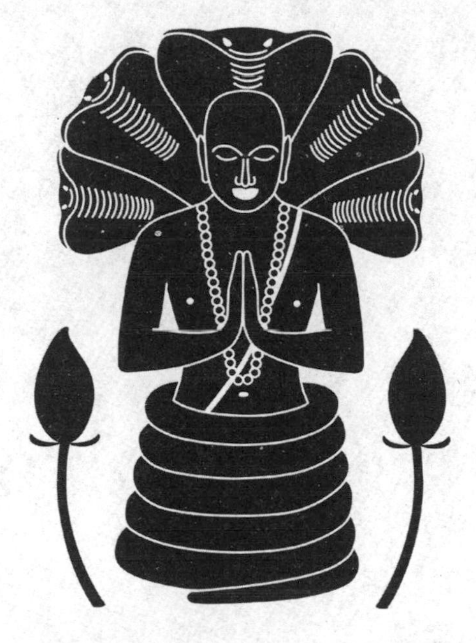

PATANJALI'S YOGA SUTRAS

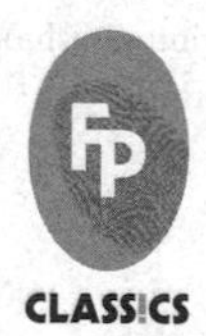

CLASSICS

Published 2023 by

FiNGERPRINT! CLASSICS
An imprint of Prakash Books India Pvt. Ltd

113/A, Darya Ganj,
New Delhi-110 002
Email: info@prakashbooks.com/sales@prakashbooks.com

facebook www.facebook.com/fingerprintpublishing
twitter www.twitter.com/FingerprintP
www.fingerprintpublishing.com

ISBN: 978 93 5440 701 7

Processed & printed in India

First, we have to bear in mind that we are all debtors to the world and the world does not owe us anything. It is a great privilege for all of us to be allowed to do anything for the world. In helping the world we really help ourselves. The second point is that there is a God in this universe. It is not true that this universe is drifting and stands in need of help from you and me. God is ever present therein, He is undying and eternally active and infinitely watchful. When the whole universe sleeps, He sleeps not; He is working incessantly; all the changes and manifestations of the world are His. Thirdly, we ought not to hate anyone. This world will always continue to be a mixture of good and evil. Our duty is to sympathise with the weak and to love even the wrongdoer. The world is a grand moral gymnasium wherein we have all to take exercise so as to become stronger and stronger spiritually.

—Swami Ji on Karma Yoga

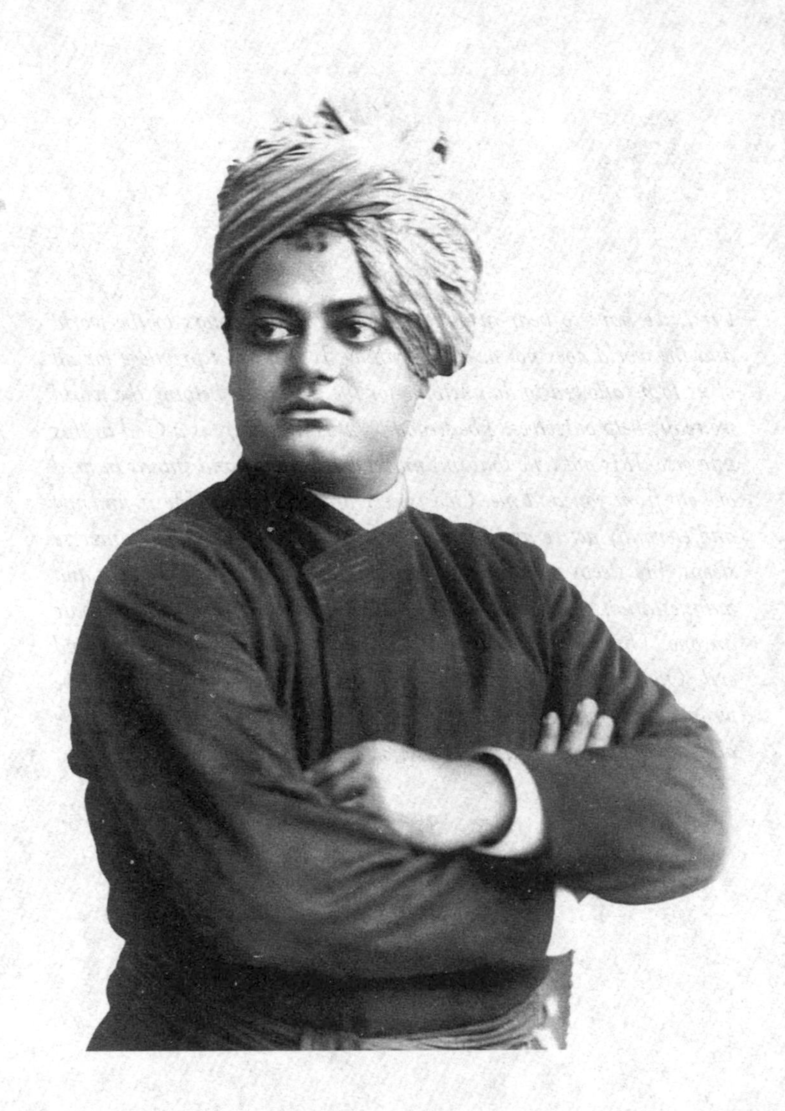

Born Narendranath Datta on January 12, 1863, in Calcutta, the capital of British India, Swami Vivekananda belonged to a traditional aristocratic Bengali Kayastha family. He was one of the nine children of Vishwanath Datta, an attorney, and Bhubaneswari Devi, a pious housewife. While his mother was religious, his father was rational and progressive.

Vivekananda, who was spiritual from a young age, was fascinated by wandering monks and used to meditate. But he was also very restive and energetic, and his mother had a hard time controlling him. From 1871 to 1877, before his family moved to Raipur, he attended Ishwar Chandra Vidyasagar's Metropolitan Institution. On his return, he joined the Presidency College in January 1880.

Vivekananda was a passionate reader. He had an appetite for subjects ranging from art, literature, philosophy, and religion to history and social science. Owing to his deep interest in Hindu mythology and Sanskrit scriptures, he read the *Ramayana,* the *Mahabharata,* the *Bhagavad Gita,* the Vedas, the Upanishads, and the Puranas. Along with being studious, he was also a sports enthusiast and took an active part in physical exercise.

Vivekananda joined Keshab Chandra Sen's social group "Nava Vidhan" where he became familiar with Western esotericism. He also became a member of the Sadharan Brahmo Samaj, a division of Brahmoism. The concepts of the Samaj shaped his beliefs. He opposed idolatry and believed in a formless God.

It was during one of his literature classes at the Scottish Church College that he learned about Ramakrishna. Vivekananda visited Dakshineswar with his friends sometime around the end of 1881 or beginning of 1882.

His meeting with Ramakrishna was a life-changing event for him.

In the beginning, he did not completely accept Ramakrishna's ideologies and even dismissed the Advaita Vedanta. But as he continued visiting him, especially after his father's death in 1884, he eventually accepted Ramakrishna as his guru, his spiritual teacher, and became his notable disciple.

Ramakrishna passed away in 1886 in Cossipore. Vivekananda, along with other disciples, set up their first monastery at Baranagar, the Ramakrishna Math. In December 1886, they all took monastic vows. It was then that he took the name "Swami Vivekananda". In the years that followed, he travelled extensively across India as a wandering monk.

During his travels, he came across people from diverse backgrounds and from various walks of life. He also familiarized himself with different social and religious customs, beliefs, and traditions. Vivekananda grew empathetic towards those who were suffering and decided to bring a change and uplift the country.

On May 31, 1893, he began his first journey abroad. He visited Japan, China, and Canada before reaching Chicago, United States, on July 30, 1893. He participated in the Parliament of World's Religions in September 1893. On the opening day, September 11, 1893, he represented India and Hinduism in his short welcome address. The speech is still remembered for its opening line—"Sisters and Brothers of America."

In the following days, he gave speeches explaining why there were disagreements between the various sects and religions. Vivekananda's "Paper on Hinduism", delivered on September 19, 1893, was an introduction to Hinduism. He enlightened the audience about the Vedanta philosophy and the concepts of god, soul, and body.

His speeches and addresses had an immediate effect not just on America, but on the whole world. He became a hero, a celebrity in no time and was reported as "the greatest figure in the Parliament of Religions" by the American newspapers. In the words of Parliament President John Henry Barrows, "India, the Mother of religions was represented by Swami Vivekananda, the Orange-monk who exercised the most wonderful influence over his auditors."

He spent the next couple of years travelling across the United States delivering lectures and speeches. In 1894, he established the Vedanta Society of New York. In 1895 and 1896, he lectured in the UK. Here, he met Margaret Elizabeth Noble (who later became Sister Nivedita) and Max Müller. He also travelled to various European countries.

Vivekananda came up with a 'four yoga' model. This included Karma Yoga, which is "purifying the mind by means of work"; Bhakti Yoga, which is "a real, genuine search after the Lord, a search beginning, continuing, and ending in love"; Rāja Yoga, which includes an interpretation of Patanjali's *Yoga Sutras*; and Jnāna Yoga, which is about realizing the truth.

He set up the Ramakrishna Mission, a twin organization of Ramakrishna Math, in Calcutta on May 1, 1897. Both the Ramakrishna Math and the Ramakrishna Mission were headquartered at Belur Math. Vivekananda also established the Advaita Ashrama in Mayavati, Uttarakhand.

In June 1899, he toured abroad with Swami Turiyananda and Sister Nivedita despite his declining health, establishing Vedanta societies in cities in the US and delivering lectures in Europe. On December 9, 1900, he came back to Calcutta.

While he continued his service and work for the Vedanta society and the Math, his health kept deteriorating. He breathed his last on July 4, 1902, while meditating. His disciples believe that he attained *mahasamadhi*.

Sangeet Kalpataru (1887), *Karma Yoga* (1896), *Rāja Yoga* (1896), *Vedanta Philosophy: An Address before the Graduate Philosophical Society* (1896), *Lectures from Colombo to Almora* (1897), *Bartaman Bharat* (1899), *Jnāna Yoga* (1899), and *My Master* (1901) and are some of his literary works published during his lifetime.

Vivekananda played a major role in introducing yoga and the Vedanta philosophies to the West. It is because of him that Hinduism gained the status of a major world religion. His birthday is observed as the National Youth Day in India, and the day he delivered his famous speech at the Parliament of World Religions, September 11, is commemorated as World Brotherhood Day.

INTRODUCTION

Before going into the *Yoga* Aphorisms I will try to discuss one great question, upon which the whole theory of religion rests, for the *Yogis.* It appears to be the consensus of the world's great minds, and it has been nearly demonstrated by researchers into physical nature, that we are the outcome and manifestation of an absolute condition, back from our current relative condition, and on our way back to that absolute. This being granted, the question is, which is better, the absolute or this state? Few people believe that this manifested state is the highest state of man. Great thinkers believe that we are manifested specimens of undifferentiated being, and this differentiated state is superior to the absolute. Because in the absolute there cannot be any quality, they imagine that it must be insensate, dull, and lifeless, that only this life can be enjoyed, and therefore we must cling to it. First of all, we want to inquire into other solutions of life. There was an old solution that man remained the same after death, that all his good sides, minus his evil sides, remained forever. Logically stated this means that man's goal is the world; this world carried a stage higher, and with elimination of its evils is the state they call heaven. This theory, on the face of it, is absurd and puerile, because it cannot be. There cannot be good without evil, or evil without good. To live in a world where all is good and there is no evil is what Sanskrit logicians call a "dream in the air." Another theory in modern times has been presented by several schools, that man's destiny is to go on improving, always struggling towards, and never reaching, the goal. This statement, though, apparently, very nice, is also absurd, because there is no such thing as motion in a straight line. Every motion is in a circle. If you could take up a stone, project it into space, and then live long enough, that stone would come back exactly to your hand. A straight line, infinitely projected, must end in a circle. Therefore, the notion that man's destiny is to progress forward and forward without ever stopping is absurd. Although extraneous to the subject, I may remark that this idea explains the ethical theory that you must not hate, and must love, because, just as in the case of electricity, or any other force, the modern theory is that the power leaves the dynamo and completes the circle back to the dynamo. So with all forces in nature; they must come back to the source. Therefore, do not hate anybody, because that force, that hatred, which comes out of you, must, in the long run, come back to you. If you love, that love will come back to you, completing the circuit. It is as certain as can be, that every bit of hatred that goes out of the heart of a man comes back to him full force; nothing can stop it, and every impulse of love comes back to him. On other and practical grounds we see that the theory of eternal progression is untenable, for destruction is the goal of everything earthly. All our struggles and hopes and fears and joys, what will they lead to? We will all end in death. Nothing is so certain as this. Where, then, is this motion in a straight line—this infinite progression? It is only going out to a distance, and again coming back to the centre from which it started. See how, from nebulæ, the sun, moon, and stars, are produced;

then they dissolve, and go back to nebulæ. The same is being done everywhere. The plant takes material from the earth, dissolves, and gives it back. Every form in this world is taken out of corresponding atoms and goes back to those atoms.

It cannot be that the same law acts differently in different places. Law is uniform. Nothing is more certain than that. If this is the law of nature, so it is with thought; it will dissolve and come back to its origin; whether we will it or not we shall have to return to the origin, which is called God or Absolute. We all came from God, and we are all bound to go back to God, call that God by any name you like; call Him God, or Absolute or Nature, or by any hundred names you like, the fact remains the same. "From whom all this universe comes out, in whom all that is born lives, and to whom all returns." This is one fact that is certain. Nature works on the same plan; what is being worked out in one sphere is being worked out in millions of spheres. What you see with the planets, the same will it be with this earth, with men and with the stars. The huge wave is a mighty compound of small waves, it may be of millions; the life of the whole world is a compound of millions of little lives, and the death of the whole world is the compound of the deaths of those millions of little beings.

Now the question arises, is going back to God the higher state, or is it not? The philosophers of the *Yoga* school answer emphatically that it is. They say that man's present state is a degeneration; that there is no one religion on the face of the earth which says that man is an improvement. The idea as that his beginning is perfect and pure, that he degenerates until he cannot degenerate further, and that there must come a time when he shoots upward again to complete the circle; the circle must be there. However low he goes, he must ultimately take the upward bend again, and go back to the original source, which is God. Man comes from God in the beginning, in the middle he becomes man, and in the end he goes back to God. This is the method of putting it in the Dualistic form. The Monistic form says that man is God, and goes back to Him again. If our present state is the higher one, then why is there so much horror and misery, and why is there an end to it? If this is the higher state, why does it end? That which corrupts and degenerates cannot be the highest state. Why should it be so diabolical, so unsatisfying? It is only excusable, inasmuch as, through it, we are taking a higher groove; we have to pass through it in order to become regenerate again. Put a seed into the ground and it disintegrates, dissolves after a time, and out of that dissolution comes the splendid tree. Every seed must degenerate to become the stately tree. So it follows that the sooner we get out of this state we call "man" the better for us. Is it by committing suicide that we get out of this state? Not at all. That will be making it all the worse. Torturing ourselves, or condemning the world, is not the way to get out. We have to pass through the "Slough of Despond," and the sooner we are through the better. But it must always be remembered that this is not the highest state.

The really difficult part to understand is that this state, the Absolute, which has been called the highest, is not, as some fear, that of the zoophite, or of the stone. That would be a dangerous thing to think. According to these thinkers there are only two states of existence, one of the stone, and the other of thought. What right have they to limit existence to these two? Is there not something infinitely superior to thought? The vibrations of light, when they are very low, we do not see; when they become a little more intense they become light to us; when they become still more intense we do not see them; it is dark to us. Is the darkness in the end the same as in the beginning? Certainly not; it is the difference of the two poles. Is the thoughtlessness of the stone the same as the thoughtlessness of God? Certainly not. God does not think; He does not reason; why should He? Is anything unknown to Him, that He should reason? The stone cannot reason; God does not. Such is the difference. These philosophers think it is awful if we go beyond thought; they find nothing beyond thought.

There are much higher states of existence beyond reasoning. It is really beyond the intellect that the first stage of religious life is to be found. When you step beyond thought and intellect and all reasoning, you make the first step towards God; and that is the beginning of life. This commonly called life is but an embryo state.

The next question will be, what proof is there that this state beyond thought and reasoning is the highest state? In the first place, all the great men of the world, much greater than those that only talk, men who moved the world, men who never thought of any selfish ends whatever, have declared that this is but a little stage on the way, that the Infinite is beyond. In the second place, they not only say so, but lay it open to everyone, they leave their methods, and all can follow in their steps. In the third place, there is no other way left. There is no other explanation. Taking for granted that there is no higher state, why are we going through this circle all the time; what reason can explain the world? The sensible will be the limit to our knowledge if we cannot go farther, if we must not ask for anything more. This is what is called agnosticism. But what reason is there to believe in the testimony of the senses? I would call that man a true agnostic who would stand still in the street and die. If reason is all in all it leaves us no place to stand on this side of nihilism. If a man is agnostic of everything, but money, fame, and name, he is only a fraud. Kant has proved beyond all doubt that we cannot penetrate beyond the tremendous dead wall called reason. But that is the very first idea upon which Indian thought takes its stand, and dares to seek, and succeeds in finding something higher than reason, where alone the explanation of the present state is to be found. This is the value of the study of something that will take us beyond the world. "Thou art our Father, and wilt take us to the other shore of this ocean of ignorance;" that is the science of religion; nothing else can be.

CONTENTS

PART I

SAMĀDHI PADA

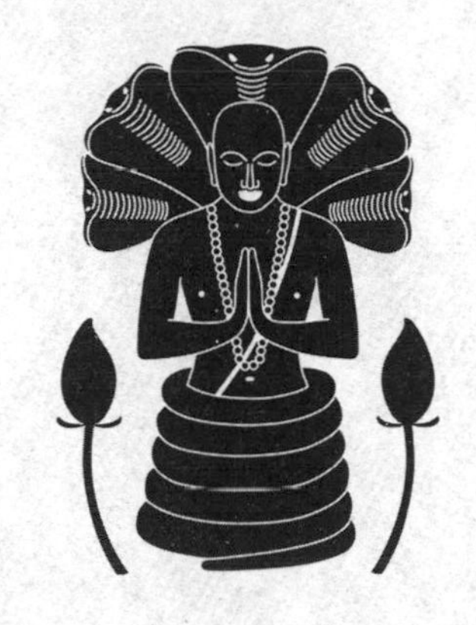

Concentration: Its Spiritual Uses

॥ प्रथमः समाधिपादः ॥

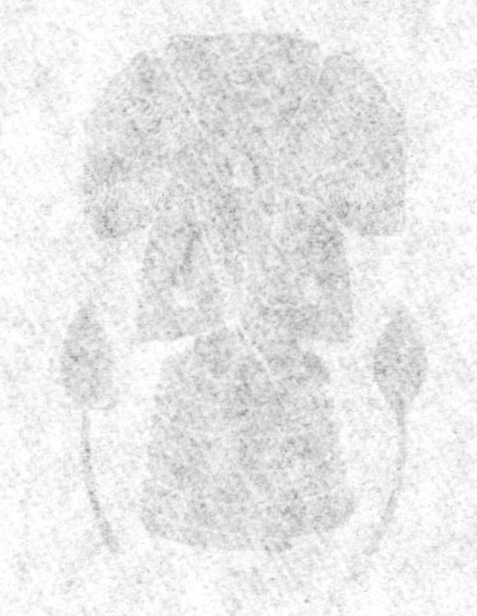

1

अथ योगानुशासनम्

atha yogānuśāsanam

Now concentration is explained.

2

योगश्चित्तवृत्तिनिरोधः

yogaś-citta-vṛtti-nirodhaḥ

Yoga is restraining the mind-stuff (Chitta) from taking various forms (Vrttis).

A good deal of explanation is necessary here. We have to understand what *Chitta* is, and what are these *Vrttis*. I have this eye. Eyes do not see. Take away the brain centre which is in the head, the eyes will still be there, the retinæ complete, and also the picture, and yet the eyes will not see. So the eyes are only a secondary instrument, not the organ of vision. The organ of vision is in the nerve centre of the brain. The two eyes will not be sufficient alone. Sometimes a man is asleep with his eyes open. The light is there and the picture is there, but a third thing is necessary; mind must be joined to the organ. The eye is the external instrument, we need also the brain centre and the agency of the mind. Carriages roll down a street and you do not hear them. Why? Because your mind has not attached itself to the organ of hearing. First there is the instrument, then there is the organ, and third, the mind attachment to these two. The mind takes the impression farther in, and presents it to the determinative faculty—*Buddhi*—which reacts. Along with this reaction flashes the idea of egoism. Then this mixture of action and reaction is presented to the *Purusa*, the real Soul, who perceives an object in this mixture. The organs (*Indriyas*), together with the mind (*Manas*), the determinative faculty (*Buddhi*) and egoism (*Ahamkara*), form the group called the *Antahkarana* (the internal instrument). They are but various processes in the mind-stuff, called *Chitta*. The waves of thought in the *Chitta* are called *Vrtti* ("the whirlpool" is the literal translation). What is thought? Thought is a force, as is gravitation or repulsion. It is absorbed from the infinite storehouse of force in nature; the instrument called *Chitta* takes hold of that force, and, when it passes out at the other end it is called thought. This force is supplied to us through food, and out of that food the body obtains the power of motion, etc. Others, the finer forces, it throws out in what we call thought. Naturally we see that the mind is not intelligent; yet it appears to be intelligent. Why? Because the intelligent soul is behind it. You are the only sentient being; mind is only the instrument through which you catch the external world. Take this book; as a book it does not exist outside, what exists outside is unknown and unknowable. It is the suggestion that gives a blow to the mind, and the mind gives out the reaction.

If a stone is thrown into the water the water is thrown against it in the form of waves. The real universe is the occasion of the reaction of the mind. A book form, or an elephant form, or a man form, is not outside; all that we know is our mental reaction from the outer suggestion. Matter is the "permanent possibility of sensation," said John Stuart Mill. It is only the suggestion that is outside. Take an oyster for example. You know how pearls are made. A grain of sand or something gets inside and begins to irritate it, and the oyster throws a sort of enamelling around the sand, and this makes the pearl. This whole universe is our own enamel, so to say, and the real universe is the grain of sand. The ordinary man will never understand it, because, when he tries to, he throws out an enamel, and sees only his own enamel. Now we understand what is meant by these *Vrttis*. The real man is behind the mind, and the mind is the instrument in his hands, and it is his intelligence that is percolating through it. It is only when you stand behind it that it becomes intelligent. When man gives it up it falls to pieces, and is nothing. So you understand what is meant by *Chitta*. It is the mind-stuff, and *Vrttis* are the waves and ripples rising in it when external causes impinge on it. These *Vrttis* are our whole universe.

The bottom of the lake we cannot see, because its surface is covered with ripples. It is only possible when the rippled have subsided, and the water is calm, for us to catch a glimpse of the bottom. If the water is muddy, the bottom will not be seen; if the water is agitated all the time, the bottom will not be seen. If the water is clear, and there are no waves, we shall see the bottom. That bottom of the lake is our own true Self; the lake is the *Chitta*, and the waves are the *Vrttis*. Again, this mind is in three states; one is darkness, which is called *Tamas*, just as in brutes and idiots; it only acts to injure others. No other idea comes into that state of mind. Then there is the active state of mind, *Rajas*, whose chief motives are power and enjoyment. "I will be powerful and rule others." Then, at last, when the waves cease, and the water of the lake becomes clear, there is the state called *Sattva*, serenity, calmness. It is not inactive, but rather intensely active. It is the greatest manifestation of power to be calm. It is easy to be active. Let the reins go, and the horses will drag you down. Anyone can do that, but he who can stop the plunging horses is the strong man. Which requires the greater strength, letting go, or restraining? The calm man is not the man who is dull. You must not mistake *Sattva* for dullness, or laziness. The calm man is the one who has restraint of these waves. Activity is the manifestation of the lower strength, calmness of the superior strength.

This *Chitta* is always trying to get back to its natural pure state, but the organs draw it out. To restrain it, and to check this outward tendency, and to start it on the return journey to that essence of intelligence is the first step in *Yoga*, because only in this way can the *Chitta* get into its proper course.

Although this *Chitta* is in every animal, from the lowest to the highest, it is only in the human form that we find intellect, and until the mind-stuff can take the form of intellect it is not possible for it to return through all these steps, and liberate the soul. Immediate salvation is impossible for the cow and the dog, although they have mind, because their *Chitta* cannot as yet take that form which we call intellect.

Chitta manifests itself in all these different forms—scattering, darkening, weakening, and concentrating. These are the four states in which the mind-stuff manifests itself. First a scattered form, is activity. Its tendency is to manifest in the form of pleasure or of pain. Then the dull form is darkness, the only tendency of which is to injure others. The commentator says the first form is natural to the *Devas*, the angels, and the second is the demoniacal form. The *Ekagra*, the concentrated form of the *Chitta*, is what brings us to *Samādhi.*

3

तदा द्रष्टुः स्वरूपेऽवस्थानम्

tadā dras.t.uh. svarūpe-'vasthānam

> At that time (the time of concentration) the seer (the Purasa) rests in his own (unmodified) state.

As soon as the waves have stopped, and the lake has become quiet, we see the ground below the lake. So with the mind; when it is calm, we see what our own nature is; we do not mix ourself but remain our own selves.

4

वृत्तिसारूप्यमितरत्र

vṛtti sārūpyam-itaratra

> At other times (other than that of concentration) the seer is identified with the modifications.

For instance, I am in a state of sorrow; someone blames me; this is a modification, *Vrtti*, and I identify myself with it, and the result is misery.

5

वृत्तयः पञ्चतय्यः क्लिष्टा अक्लिष्टाः

vṛttayaḥ pañcatayyaḥ kliṣṭākliṣṭāḥ

There are five classes of modification, painful and not painful.

6

प्रमाणविपर्ययविकल्पनिद्रास्मृतयः

pramāṇa-viparyaya-vikalpa-
nidrā-smṛtayaḥ

(These are) right knowledge, indiscrimination, verbal delusion, sleep, and memory.

7

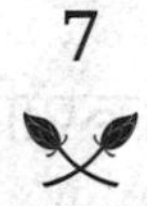

प्रत्यक्षानुमानागमाः प्रमाणानि

pratyakṣānumānāgamāḥ pramāṇāni

Direct perception, inference, and competent evidence, are proofs.

When two of our perceptions do not contradict each other we call it proof. I hear something, and, if it contradicts something already perceived, I begin to fight it out, and do not believe it. There are also three kinds of proof. Direct perception, *Pratyaksham*, whatever we see and feel, is proof, if there has been nothing to delude the senses. I see the world; that is sufficient proof that it exists. Secondly, *Anumāna*, inference; you see a sign, and from the sign you come to the thing signified. Thirdly, *Āptavakyam*, the direct perception of the *Yogi*, of those who have seen the truth. We are all of us struggling towards knowledge, but you and I have to struggle hard, and come to knowledge through a long tedious process of reasoning, but the *Yogi*, the pure one, has gone beyond all this. Before his mind, the past, the present, and the future, are alike one book for him to read; he does not require to go through all this tedious process, and his words are proofs, because he sees knowledge in himself; he is the Omniscient One. These, for instance, are the authors of the Sacred Scriptures; therefore the Scriptures are proof, and, if any such persons are living now, their words will be proof. Other philosophers go into long discussions about this *Āpta*, and they say, what is the proof that this is truth? The proof is because they see it; because whatever I see is proof, and whatever you see is proof, if it does not contradict any past knowledge. There is knowledge beyond the senses, and whenever it does not contradict reason and past human experience, that knowledge is proof. Any madman may come into this room and say that he sees angels around him, that would not be proof. In the first place it must be true knowledge, and, secondly, it must not contradict knowledge of the past, and thirdly, it must depend upon the character of the man. I hear it said that the character of the man is not of so much importance as what he may say; we must first hear what he says. This may be true in other things; a man may be wicked, and yet make an astronomical discovery, but in religion it is different, because no impure man will ever have the power to reach the truths of religion. Therefore, we have first of all to see that the man who declares himself to be an *Āpta* is a perfectly unselfish and holy person; secondly that he has reached beyond the senses, and thirdly that what he says does not contradict the past knowledge of humanity. Any new discovery of truth does not contradict the past truth, but fits into it. And, fourthly, that truth must have a possibility of verification. If a man says "I have seen a vision," and tells me that I have no right to see it, I believe him not. Everyone must have the power to see it for himself. No one who sells his knowledge is an *Āpta.* All these conditions must be fulfilled; you must first see that the man is pure, and that he has no selfish motive; that he has no thirst for gain or fame. Secondly, he must show that he is superconscious. He must have given us something that we cannot get from our senses, and which is for benefit of the world. Thirdly, we must see that it does not contradict other truths; if it contradicts other scientific truths reject it at once. Fourthly, the man should never be singular; he should only represent what all men can attain. The three sorts of proof, are, then, direct sense perception, inference, and the words of an *Āpta.* I cannot translate this word into English. It is not the word inspired, because that comes from outside, while this comes from himself. The literal meaning is "attained."

8

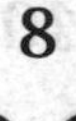

विपर्ययो मिथ्याज्ञानमतद्रूपप्रतिष्ठम्

viparyayo mithyājñānam-atad-rūpa-pratiṣṭham

> Indiscrimination is false knowledge not established in real nature.

The next class of *Vrttis* that arise is mistaking the one thing for another, as a piece of mother-of-pearl is taken for a piece of silver.

9

शब्दज्ञानानुपाति वस्तुशून्यो विकल्पः

śabda-jñānānupātī vastu-śūnyo vikalpaḥ

> Verbal delusion follows from words having no (corresponding) reality.

There is another class of *Vrttis* called *Vikalpa*. A word is uttered, and we do not wait to consider its meaning; we jump to a conclusion immediately. It is the sign of weakness of the *Chitta*. Now you can understand the theory of restraint. The weaker the man the less he has of restraint. Consider yourselves always in that way. When you are going to be angry or miserable, reason it out, how it is that some news that has come to you is throwing your mind into *Vrttis*.

10

अभाव प्रत्ययालम्बना वृत्तिर्निद्रा

abhāva pratyayālambanā tamo-vṛttir-nidra

Sleep is a *Vrtti* which embraces the feeling of voidness.

The next class of *Vrttis* is called sleep and dream. When we awake we know that we have been sleeping; we can only have memory of perception. That which we do not perceive we never can have any memory of. Every reaction is a wave in the lake. Now, if, during sleep, the mind has no waves, it would have no perceptions, positive or negative, and, therefore, we would not remember them. The very reason of our remembering sleep is that during sleep there was a certain class of waves in the mind. Memory is another class of *Vrttis*, which is called *Smrti*.

11

अनुभूतविषयासम्प्रमोषः स्मृतिः

anubhūta-viṣayāsaṁpramoṣaḥ smṛtiḥ

Memory is when the (Vrttis of) perceived subjects do not slip away (and through impressions come back to consciousness).

Memory can be caused by the previous three. For instance, you hear a word. That word is like a stone thrown into the lake of the *Chitta*; it causes a ripple, and that ripple rouses a series of ripples; this is memory. So in sleep. When the peculiar kind of ripple called sleep throws the *Chitta* into a ripple of memory it is called a dream. Dream is another form of the ripple which in the waking state is called memory.

12

अभ्यासवैराग्याभ्यां तन्निरोधः

abhyāsa-vairāgyābhyāṃ tan-nirodhaḥ

Their control is by practice and non-attachment.

The mind, to have this non-attachment, must be clear, good and rational. Why should we practice? Because each action is like the pulsations quivering over the surface of the lake. The vibration dies out, and what is left? The *Samsharas*, the impressions. When a large number of these impressions is left on the mind they coalesce, and become a habit. It is said "habit is second nature;" it is first nature also, and the whole nature of man; everything that we are, is the result of habit. That gives us consolation, because, if it is only habit, we can make and unmake it at any time. The *Samshara* is left by these vibrations passing out of our mind, each one of them leaving its result. Our character is the sum-total of these marks, and according as some particular wave prevails one takes that tone. If good prevail one becomes good, if wickedness one wicked, if joyfulness one becomes happy. The only remedy for bad habits is counter habits; all the bad habits that have left their impressions are to be controlled by good habits. Go on doing good, thinking holy thoughts continuously; that is the only way to suppress base impressions. Never say any man is hopeless, because he only represents a character, a bundle of habits, and these can be checked by new and better ones. Character is repeated habits, and repeated habits alone can reform character.

13

तत्र स्थितौ यत्नोऽभ्यासः

tatra sthitau yatno'bhyāsaḥ

Continuous struggle to keep them (the *Vrttis*) perfectly restrained is practice.

What is this practice? The attempt to restrain the mind in the *Chitta* form, to prevent its going out into waves.

14

स तु दीर्घकालनैरन्तर्यसत्कारासेवितो दृढभूमिः

sa tu dīrgha-kāla-nairantarya-satkārāsevito drdha-bhūmiḥ

Its ground becomes firm by long, constant efforts with great love (for the end to be attained).

Restraint does not come in one day, but by long continued practice.

15

दृष्टानुश्रविकविषयवितृष्णस्य वशीकारसंज्ञा वैराग्यम्

dṛṣṭānuśravika-viṣaya-vitṛṣṇasya vaśīkāra-saṃjnā vairāgyam

> That effort, which comes to those who have given up their thirst after objects either seen or heard, and which wills to control the objects, is non-attachment.

Two motives of our actions are (1) What we see ourselves; (2) The experience of others. These two forces are throwing the mind, the lake, into various waves. Renunciation is the power of battling against these, and holding the mind in check. Renunciation of these two motives is what we want. I am passing through a street, and a man comes and takes my watch. That is my own experience. I see it myself, and it immediately throws my *Chitta* into a wave, taking the form of anger. Allow that not to come. If you cannot prevent that, you are nothing; if you can, you have *Vairāgyam.* Similarly, the experience of the worldly-minded teaches us that sense enjoyments are the highest ideal. These are tremendous temptations. To deny them, and not allow the mind to come into a wave form with regard to them is renunciation; to control the twofold motive powers arising from my own experience, and from the experience of others, and thus prevent the *Chitta* from being governed by them, is *Vairāgyam*. These should be controlled by me, and not I by them. This sort of mental strength is called renunciation. This *Vairāgyam* is the only way to freedom.

16

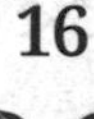

तत्परं पुरुषख्यातेर्गुणवैतृष्ण्यम्

tat-paraṃ puruṣa-khyāter guṇa-vaitṛṣṇyam

> That extreme non-attachment, giving up even the qualities, shows (the real nature of) the *Purusa*.

It is the highest manifestation of power when it takes away even our attraction towards the qualities. We have first to understand what the *Purusa*, the Self, is, and what are the qualities. According to *Yoga* philosophy the whole of nature consists of three qualities; one is called *Tamas*, another *Rajas* and the third *Sattva*. These three qualities manifest themselves in the physical world as attraction, repulsion, and control. Everything that is in nature, all these manifestations, are combinations and recombinations of these three forces. This nature has been divided into various categories by the *Sānkhyas*; the Self of man is beyond all these, beyond nature. It is effulgent, pure and perfect. Whatever of intelligence we see in nature is but the reflection from this Self upon nature. Nature itself is insentient. You must remember that the word nature also includes the mind; mind is in nature; thought is in nature; from thought, down to the grossest form of matter, everything is in nature, the manifestation of nature. This nature has covered the Self of man, and when nature takes away the covering the Self becomes unveiled, and appears in its own glory. This non-attachment, as it is described in Aphorism 15 (as being control of nature) is the greatest help towards manifesting the Self. The next aphorism defines *Samādhi*, perfect concentration, which is the goal of the *Yogi*.

17

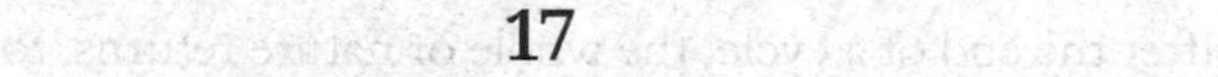

वितर्कविचारानन्दास्मितारूपानुगमात् सम्प्रज्ञातः

vitarka-vicārānandāsmitā-rupānugamāt saṁprajñātaḥ

> The concentration called right knowledge is that which is followed by reasoning, discrimination, bliss, unqualified ego.

This *Samādhi* is divided into two varieties. One is called the *Samprajnāta*, and the other the *Asamprajnāta*. The *Samprajnāta* is of four varieties. In this *Samādhi* come all the powers of controlling nature. The first variety is called the *Savitarka*, when the mind meditates upon an object again and again, by isolating it from other objects. There are two sorts of objects for meditation, the categories of nature, and the *Purusa*. Again, the categories are of two varieties; the twenty-four categories are insentient, and the one sentient is the *Purusa*. When the mind thinks of the elements of nature by thinking of their beginning and their end, this is one sort of *Savitarka*.

The words require explanation. This part of *Yoga* is based entirely on *Sānkhya* Philosophy, about which I have already told you. As you will remember, egoism and will, and mind, have a common basis, and that common basis is called the *Chitta*, the mind-stuff, out of which they are all manufactured. This mind-stuff takes in the forces of nature, and projects them as thought. There must be something, again, where both force and matter are one. This is called *Avyakta*, the unmanifested state of nature before creation, and to which, after the end of a cycle, the whole of nature returns, to again come out after another period. Beyond that is the *Purusa*, the essence of intelligence. There is no liberation in getting powers. It is a worldly search after enjoyment in this life; all search for enjoyment is vain; this is the old, old lesson which man finds it so hard to learn. When he does learn it, he gets out of the universe and becomes free. The possession of what are called occult powers is only intensifying the world, and in the end intensifying suffering. Though, as a scientist, Patanjali is bound to point out the possibilities of this science, he never misses an opportunity to warn us against these powers. Knowledge is power, and as soon as we begin to know a thing we get power over it; so also, when the mind begins to meditate on the different elements it gains power over them. That sort of meditation where the external gross elements are the objects is called *Savitarka*. *Vitarka* means question, *Savitarka* with question, questioning the elements, as it were, that they may give up their truths and their powers to the man who meditates upon them. Again, in the very same meditation, when one struggles to take the elements out of time and space, and think of them as they are, it is called *Nirvitarka*, without question. When the meditation goes a step higher, and takes the *Tanmātras* as its object, and thinks of them as in time and space, it is called *Savichāra*, with discrimination, and when in the same meditation one gets beyond time and space, and thinks of the fine elements as they are, it is called *Nirvichāra*, without discrimination. The next step is when the elements are given up, either as gross or as fine, and the object of meditation is the interior organ, the thinking organ, and when the thinking organ is thought of as bereft of the qualities of activity, and of dullness, it is then called *Sānanda*, the blissful *Samādhi*. When the mind itself is the object of meditation, when meditation become very ripe and concentrated, when all ideas of the gross materials, or fine materials, when the *Sattva* state only of the Ego remains, but differentiated from all other objects, it is called *Asmitā Samādhi*. The man who has attained to this has attained to what is called in the *Vedas* "bereft of body." He can think of himself as without his gross body; but he will have to think of himself as with a fine body. Those that in this state get merged in nature without attaining the goal are called *Prakrtilayas*, but those who do not even stop even there reach the goal, which is freedom.

18

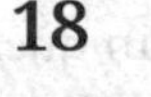

विरामप्रत्ययाभ्यासपूर्वः संस्कारशेषोऽन्यः

virāma-pratyayābhyāsa-pūrvaḥ saṃskāra-śeṣo'nyaḥ

There is another *Samādhi* which is attained by the constant practice of cessation of all mental activity, in which the *Chitta* retains only the unmanifested impressions.

This is the perfect superconscious *Asamprajnāta Samādhi*, the state which gives us freedom. The first state does not give us freedom, does not liberate the soul. A man may attain to all powers, and yet fall again. There is no safeguard until the soul goes beyond nature, and beyond conscious concentration. It is very difficult to attain, although its method seems very easy. Its method is to hold the mind as the object, and whenever through comes, to strike it down, allowing no thought to come into the mind, thus making it an entire vacuum. When we can really do this, in that moment we shall attain liberation. When persons without training and preparation try to make their minds vacant they are likely to succeed only in covering themselves with *Tamas*, material of ignorance, which makes the mind dull and stupid, and leads them to think that they are making a vacuum of the mind. To be able to really do that is a manifestation of the greatest strength, of the highest control. When this state, *Asamprajnāta*, superconsciousness, is reached, the *Samādhi* becomes seedless. What is meant by that? In that sort of concentration when there is consciousness, where the mind has succeeded only in quelling the waves in the *Chitta* and holding them down, they are still there in the form of tendencies, and these tendencies (or seeds) will become waves again, when the time comes. But when you have destroyed all these tendencies, almost destroyed the mind, then it has become seedless, there are no more seeds in the mind out of which to manufacture again and again this plant of life, this ceaseless round of birth and death. You may ask, what state would that be, in which we should have no knowledge? What we call knowledge is a lower state than the one beyond knowledge. You must always bear in mind that the extremes look very much the same. The low vibration of light is darkness, and the very high vibration of light is darkness also, but one is real darkness, and the other is really intense light; yet their appearance is the same. So, ignorance is the lowest state, knowledge is the middle state, and beyond knowledge is a still higher state. Knowledge itself is a manufactured something, a combination; it is not reality. What will be the result of constant practice of this higher concentration? All old tendencies of restlessness, and dullness, will be destroyed, as well as the tendencies of goodness too. It is just the same as with the metals that are used with gold to takc off the dirt and alloy. When the ore is smelted down, the dross is burnt along with the alloy. So this constant controlling power will stop the previous bad tendencies and, eventually, the good ones also. Those good and evil tendencies will suppress each other, and there will remain the Soul, in all its glorious splendour, untrammelled by either good or bad, and that Soul is omnipresent, omnipotent, and omniscient. By giving up all powers it has become omnipotent, by giving up all life it is beyond mortality; it has become life itself. Then the Soul will know it neither had birth nor death, neither want of heaven nor of earth. It will know that it neither came nor went; it was nature which was moving, and that movement was reflected upon the Soul. The form of the light is moving, it is reflected and cast by the camera upon the wall, and the wall foolishly thinks it is moving. So with all of us: it is the *Chitta* constantly moving, manipulating itself into various forms, and we think that we are these various forms. All these delusions will vanish. When that free Soul will command—not pray or beg, but command—then whatever It desires will be immediately fulfilled; whatever

It wants It will be able to do. According to the *Sānkhya* Philosophy there is no God. It says that there cannot be any God of this universe, because if there were He must be a Soul, and a Soul must be one of two things, either bound or free. How can the soul that is bound by nature, or controlled by nature, create? It is itself a slave. On the other hand, what business has the soul that is free to create and manipulate all these things? It has no desires, so cannot have any need to create. Secondly, it says the theory of God is an unnecessary one; nature explains all. What is the use of any God? But *Kapila* teaches that there are many souls, who, through nearly attaining perfection, fall short because they cannot perfectly renounce all powers. Their minds for a time merge in nature, to re-emerge as its masters. We shall all become such gods, and, according to the *Sānkhyas*, the God spoken of in the *Vedas* really means one of these free souls. Beyond them there is not an eternally free and blessed Creator of the universe. On the other hand the *Yogis* say, "Not so, there is a God; there is one Soul separate from all other souls, and He is the eternal Master of all creation, the Ever Free, the Teacher of all teachers." The *Yogis* admit that those the *Sānkhyas* called "merged in nature" also exist. They are *Yogis* who have fallen short of perfection, and though, for a time debarred from attaining the goal, remain as rulers of parts of the universe.

19

भवप्रत्ययो विदेहप्रकृतिलयानाम्

bhava-pratyayo videha-prakṛti-layānām

(This *Samādhi*, when not followed by extreme non-attachment) becomes the cause of the re-manifestation of the gods and of those that become merged in nature.

The gods in the Indian systems represent certain high offices which are being filled successively by various souls. But none of them is perfect.

20

श्रद्धावीर्यस्मृतिसमाधिप्रज्ञापूर्वक इतरेषाम्

śraddhā-vīrya-smṛti-samādhi-prajñā-pūrvaka itareṣām

To others (this Samādhi) comes through faith, energy, memory, concentration, and discrimination of the real.

These are they who do not want the position of gods, or even that of rulers of cycles. They attain to liberation.

21

तीव्रसंवेगानामासन्नः

tīvra-saṃvegānām-āsannaḥ

Success is speedy for the extremely energetic.

22

मृदुमध्याधिमात्रत्वात्ततोऽपि विशेषः

mṛdu-madhyādhimātratvāt-tato'pi viśeṣaḥ

The success of Yogis differs according to whether the means they adopt are mild, medium or intense.

23

ईश्वरप्रणिधानाद्वा

īśvara-praṇidhānād-vā

Or by devotion to *Isvara.*

24

क्लेशकर्मविपाकाशयैरपरामृष्टः पुरुषविशेष ईश्वरः

kleśa-karma-vipākāśayair-aparāmṛṣṭaḥ
puruṣa-viśeṣa Īśvaraḥ

Isvara (the Supreme Ruler) is a special *Purusa*, untouched by misery, the results of actions, or desires.

We must again remember that this Patanjali *Yoga* Philosophy is based upon that of the *Sānkhyas*, only that in the latter there is no place for God, while with the *Yogis* God has a place. The *Yogis*, however, avoid many ideas about God, such as creating. God as the Creator of the Universe is not meant by the *Isvara* of the *Yogis*, although, according to the *Vedas*, *Isvara* is the Creator of the universe. Seeing that the universe is harmonious, it must be the manifestation of one will. The *Yogis* and *Sānkhyas* both avoid the question of creation. The *Yogis* want to establish a God, but carefully avoid this question; they do not raise it at all. Yet you will find that they arrive at God in a peculiar fashion of their own. They say:

25

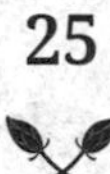

तत्र निरतिशयं सर्वज्ञत्वबीजम्

tatra niratiśayaṃ sarvajñatva-bījam

In Him becomes infinite that all-knowingness which in others is (only) a germ.

The mind must always travel between two extremes. You can think of limited space, but the very idea of that gives you also unlimited space. Close your eyes and think of a little space, and at the same time that you perceive the little circle, you have a circle round it of unlimited dimensions. It is the same with time. Try to think of a second, you will have, with the same act of perception, to think of time which is unlimited. So with knowledge. Knowledge is only a germ in man, but you will have to think of infinite knowledge around it, so that the very nature of your constitution shows us that there is unlimited knowledge, and the *Yogis* call that unlimited knowledge God.

26

स पूर्वेषामपि गुरुः कालेनानवच्छेदात्

sa eṣa pūrveṣām-api guruḥ kālenānavacchedāt

> He is the Teacher of even the ancient teachers,
> being not limited by time.

It is true that all knowledge is within ourselves, but this has to be called forth by another knowledge. Although the capacity to know is inside us, it must be called out, and that calling out of knowledge can only be got, a *Yogi* maintains, through another knowledge. Dead, insentient matter, never calls out knowledge. It is the action of knowledge that brings out knowledge. Knowing beings must be with us to call forth what is in us, so these teachers were always necessary. The world was never without them, and no knowledge can come without them. God is the Teacher of all teachers, because these teachers, however great they may have been—gods or angels—were all bound and limited by time, and God is not limited by time. These are the two peculiar distinctions of the *Yogis*. The first is that in thinking of the limited, the mind must think of the unlimited, and that if one part of the perception is true the other must be, for the reason that their value as perceptions of the mind is equal. The very fact that man has a little knowledge, shows that God has unlimited knowledge. If I am to take one, why not the other? Reason forces me to take both or reject both. If I believe that there is a man with a little knowledge, I must also admit that there is someone behind him with unlimited knowledge. The second deduction is that no knowledge can come without a teacher. It is true as the modern philosophers say, that there is something in man which evolves out of him; all knowledge is in man, but certain environments are necessary to call it out. We cannot find any knowledge without teacher, if there are men teachers, god teachers, or angel teachers, they are all limited; who was the teacher before them? We are forced to admit, as a last conclusion, One Teacher, who is not limited by time, and that One Teacher or infinite knowledge, without beginning or end, is called God.

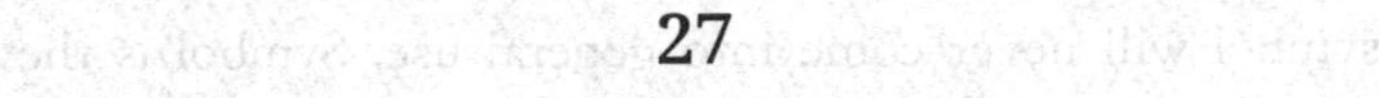

27

तस्य वाचकः प्रणवः

tasya vācakaḥ praṇavaḥ

His manifesting word is *Om.*

Every idea that you have in the mind has a counterpart in a word; the word and the thought are inseparable. The external part of the thought is what we call word, and the internal part is what we call thought. No man can, by analysis, separate thought from word. The idea that language was created by men—certain men sitting together and deciding on words, has been proved to be wrong. So long as things have existed there have been words and language. What is the connection between an idea and a word? Although we see that there must always be a word with a thought, it is not necessary that the same thought requires the same word. The thought may be the same in twenty different countries, yet the language is different. We must have a word to express each thought, but these words need not necessarily have the same sound. Sounds will vary in different nations. Our commentator says "Although the relation between thought and word is perfectly natural, yet it does not mean a rigid connection between one sound and one idea." These sounds vary, yet the relation between the sounds and the thoughts is a natural one. The connection between thoughts and sounds is good only if there be a real connection between the thing signified and the symbol, and until then that symbol will never come into general use. Symbol is the manifestor of the thing signified, and if the thing signified has already existence, and if, by experience, we know that the symbol has expressed that thing many times, then we are sure that there is the real relation between them. Even if the things are not present, there will be thousands who will know them by their symbols. There must be a natural connection between the symbol and the thing signified; then, when that symbol is pronounced, it recalled the thing signified. The commentator says the manifesting word of God is *Om*. Why does he emphasise this? There are hundreds of words for God. One thought is connected with a thousand words; the idea, God, is connected with hundreds of words, and each one stands as a symbol for God. Very good. But there must be a generalisation among all these words, some substratum, some common ground of all these symbols, and that symbol which is the common symbol will be the best, and will really be the symbol of all. In making a sound we use the larynx, and the palate as a sounding board. Is there any material sound of which all other sounds must be manifestations, one which is the most natural sound? *Om* (*Aum*) is such a sound, the basis of all sounds. The first letter, A, is the root sound, the key, pronounced without touching any part of the tongue or palate; M represents the last sound in the series, being produced by the closed lip, and the U rolls from the very root to the end of the sounding board of the mouth. Thus, *Om* represents the whole phenomena of sound producing. As such, it must be the natural symbol, the matrix of all the variant sounds. It denotes the whole range and possibility of all the words that can be made. Apart from these speculations we see that around this word *Om* are centred all the different religious ideas in India; all the various religious ideas of the *Vedas* have gathered themselves round this word *Om*. What has that to do with America and England, or any other country? Simply that the word has been retained at every stage of religious growth in India, and it has been manipulated to mean all the various ideas about God. Monists, Dualists, Mono-Dualists, Separatists, and even Atheists, took up this *Om*. *Om* has become the one symbol for the religious aspiration of the vast majority of human beings. Take, for instance, the English word God. It conveys only a limited function, and if you go beyond it, you have to add adjectives, to make it Personal, or Impersonal, or Absolute God. So with the words for God in every other language; their signification is very small. This word *Om*, however, has around it all the various significances. As such it should be accepted by everyone.

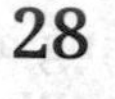

28

तज्जपस्तदर्थभावनम्

taj-japas-tad-artha-bhāvanam

> The repetition of this (Om) and meditating on its meaning (is the way).

Why should there be repetition? We have not forgotten that theory of *Samskāras*, that the sum-total of impressions lives in the mind. Impressions live in the mind, the sum-total of impressions, and they become more and more latent, but remain there, and as soon as they get the right stimulus they come out. Molecular vibration will never cease. When this universe is destroyed all the massive vibrations disappear, the sun, moon, stars, and earth, will melt down, but the vibrations must remain in the atoms. Each atom will perform the same function as the big worlds do. So the vibrations of this *Chitta* will subside, but will go on like molecular vibrations, and when they get the impulse will come out again. We can now understand what is meant by repetition. It is the greatest stimulus that can be given to the spiritual *Samskāras*. "One moment of company with the Holy makes a ship to cross this ocean of life." Such is the power of association. So this repetition of *Om*, and thinking of its meaning, is keeping good company in your own mind. Study, and then meditate and meditate, when you have studied. The light will come to you, the Self will become manifest.

But one must think of this *Om*, and of its meaning too. Avoid evil company, because the scars of old wounds are in you, and this evil company is just the heat that is necessary to call them out. In the same way we are told that good company will call out the good impressions that are in us, but which have become latent. There is nothing holier in this world than to keep good company, because the good impressions will have this same tendency to come to the surface.

29

ततः प्रत्यक्चेतनाधिगमोऽप्यन्तरायाभावश्च

tataḥ pratyak-cetanādhigamo'pyantarāyābhavaś-ca

From that is gain (the knowledge of) introspection, and the destruction of obstacles.

The first manifestation of this repetition and thinking of *Om* will be that the introspective power will be manifested more and more, and all the mental and physical obstacles will begin to vanish. What are the obstacles to the *Yogi*?

30

व्याधिस्त्यानसंशयप्रमादालस्याविरतिभ्रान्तिदर्शनालब्ध भूमिकत्वानवस्थितत्वानि चित्तविक्षेपास्तेऽन्तरायाः

vyādhi-styāna-saṃśaya-pramādālasyāvirati-bhrānti-darśanālabdha-bhūmikatvānavasthitatvāni cittavikṣepās-teantarāyāḥ

> Disease, mental laziness, doubt, calmness, cessation, false perception, non-attaining concentration, and falling away from the state when obtained, are the obstructing distractions.

Disease. This body is the boat which will carry us to the other shore of the ocean of life. It must be taken care of. Unhealthy persons cannot be *Yogis*. Mental laziness makes us lose all lively interest in the subject, without which there will neither be the will nor the energy to practice. Doubts will arise in the mind about the truth of the science, however strong one's intellectual conviction may be, until certain peculiar psychic experiences come, as hearing, or seeing, at a distance, etc.

These glimpses strengthen the mind and make the student persevere. Falling away . . . when attained. Some days or weeks when you are practising the mind will be calm and easily concentrated, and you will find yourself progressing fast. All of a sudden the progress will stop one day, and you will find yourself, as it were, stranded. Persevere. All progress proceeds by rise and fall.

31

दुःख दौर्मनस्याङ्गमेजयत्वश्वासप्रश्वासा विक्षेपसहभुवः

duḥkha daurmanasyāṅgam-ejayatva-śvāsa-praśvāsāḥ vikṣepa-sahabhuvaḥ

Grief, mental distress, tremor of the body and irregular breathing, accompany non-retention of concentration.

Concentration will bring perfect repose to mind and body every time it is practised. When the practice has been misdirected, or not enough controlled, these disturbances come. Repetition of *Om* and self-surrender to the Lord will strengthen the mind, and bring fresh energy. The nervous shakings will come to almost everyone. Do not mind them at all, but keep on practising. Practice will cure them, and make the seat firm.

32

तत्प्रतिषेधार्थमेकतत्त्वाभ्यासः

tat-pratiṣedhārtham eka-tattvābhyāsaḥ

To remedy this practice of one subject (should be made).

Making the mind take the form of one object for some time will destroy these obstacles. This is general advice. In the following aphorisms it will be expanded and particularised. As one practice cannot suit everyone, various methods will be advanced, and everyone by actual experience will find out that which helps him most.

33

मैत्रीकरुणामुदितोपेक्षाणां सुखदुःखपुण्यापुण्यविषयाणां भावनातश्चित्तप्रसादनम्

maitrī-karuṇā-muditopekṣāṇāṃ sukha-duḥkha-puṇyāpuṇya-viṣayāṇāṃ bhāvanātaś-citta-prasādanam

> Friendship, mercy, gladness, indifference, being thought of in regard to subjects, happy, unhappy, good and evil respectively, pacify the Chitta.

We must have these four sorts of ideas. We must have friendship for all; we must be merciful towards those that are in misery; when people are happy we ought to be happy, and to the wicked we must be indifferent. So with all subjects that come before us. If the subject is a good one, we shall feel friendly towards it; if the subject of thought is one that is miserable we must be merciful towards the subject. If it is good we must be glad, if it is evil we must be indifferent. These attitudes of the mind towards the different subjects that come before it will make the mind peaceful. Most of our difficulties in our daily lives come from being unable to hold our minds in this way. For instance, if a man does evil to us, instantly we want to react evil, and every reaction of evil shows that we are not able to hold the *Chitta* down; it comes out in waves towards the object, and we lose our power. Every reaction in the form of hatred or evil is so much loss to the mind, and every evil thought or deed of hatred, or any thought of reaction, if it is controlled, will be laid in our favour. It is not that we lose by thus restraining ourselves; we are gaining infinitely more than we suspect. Each time we suppress hatred, or a feeling of anger, it is so much good energy stored up in our favour; that piece of energy will be converting into the higher powers.

34

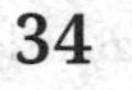

प्रच्छर्दनविधारणाभ्यां वा प्राणस्य

pracchardana-vidhāraṇābhyāṃ vā prāṇasya

By throwing out and restraining the Breath.

The word used is *Prāna*. *Prāna* is not exactly breath. It is the name for the energy that is in the universe. Whatever you see in the universe, whatever moves or works, or has life, is a manifestation of this *Prāna*. The sum-total of the energy displayed in the universe is called *Prāna*. This *Prāna*, before a cycle begins, remains in an almost motionless state, and when the cycle begins this *Prāna* begins to manifest itself. It is this *Prāna* that is manifested as motion, as the nervous motion in human beings or animals, and the same *Prāna* is manifesting as thought, and so on. The whole universe is a combination of *Prāna* and *Ākāsa*; so is the human body. Out of *Ākāsa* you get the different materials that you feel, and see, and out of *Prāna* all the various forces. Now this throwing out and restraining the *Prāna* is what is called *Prānāyāma*. Patanjali, the father of the *Yoga* Philosophy, does not give many particular directions about *Prānāyāma*, but later on other *Yogis* found out various things about this *Prānāyāma*, and made of it a great science. With Patanjali it is one of the many ways, but he does not lay much stress on it. He means that you simply throw the air out, and draw it in, and hold it for some time, that is all, and by that, the mind will become a little calmer. But, later on, you will find that out of this is evolved a particular science called *Prānāyāma*. We will hear a little of what these later *Yogis* have to say. Some of this I have told you before, but a little repetition will serve to fix it in your minds. First, you must remember that this *Prāna* is not the breath. But that which causes the motion of the breath, that which is the vitality of the breath is the *Prāna*. Again, the word *Prāna* is used of all the senses; they are all called *Prāna*, the mind is called *Prāna*; and so we see that *Prāna* is the name of a certain force. And yet we cannot call it force, because force is only the manifestation of it. It is that which manifests itself as force and everything else in the way of motion. The *Chitta*, the mind-stuff, is the engine which draws in the *Prāna* from the surroundings, and manufactures out of this *Prāna* the various vital forces—those that keep the body in preservation—and thought, will, and all other powers. By this process of breathing we can control all the various motions in the body, and the various nerve currents that are running through the body. First we begin to recognise them, and then we slowly get control over them. Now these later *Yogis* consider that there are three main currents of this *Prāna* in the human body. One they call *Idā*, another *Pingalā*, and the third *Susumnā*. *Pingalā*, according to them, is on the right side of the spinal column, and the *Idā* is on the left side, and in the middle of this spinal column is the *Susumnā*, a vacant channel. *Idā* and *Pingalā*, according to them, are the currents working in every man, and through these currents, we are performing all the functions of life. *Susumnā* is present in all, as a possibility; but it works only in the *Yogi*. You must remember that the *Yogi* changes his body; as you go on practising your body changes; it is not the same body that you had before the practice. That is very rational, and can be explained, because every new thought that we have must make, as it were, a new channel through the brain, and that explains the tremendous conservatism of human nature. Human nature likes to run through the ruts that are already there, because it is easy. If we think, just for example's sake, that the mind is like a needle, and the brain substance a soft lump before it, then each thought that we have makes a street, as it were, in the brain, and this street would close up, but that the grey matter comes and makes a lining to keep it separate. If there were no grey matter there would be no memory, because memory means going over these old streets, retracing a thought as it were. Now perhaps you have remarked that when I talk on subjects that in which I take a few ideas that are familiar to everyone, and combine, and recombine them, it is easy to follow, because these channels are present in everyone's brain, and it is only necessary to recur to them. But whenever a new subject comes new channels have to be made, so it is not understood so readily. And that is why the brain (it is the brain, and not the people themselves) refuses unconsciously to be acted upon by new ideas. It resists. The *Prāna* is trying to make new channels, and the brain will not allow it. This is the secret of conservatism. The less channels there have been in the brain, and the less the needle of the *Prāna* has made these passages, the more conservative will be the brain, the more it will struggle against new thoughts. The more thoughtful the mane, the more complicated will be the streets in his brain, and the more easily he will take to new ideas, and understand them. So with every fresh idea; we make a new impression in the brain, cut new channels though the brain-stuff, and that is why we find that in the practice of *Yoga* (it being an entirely new set of thoughts and motives) there is so much physical resistance at first. That is why we find that the part of religion which deals with the world side of nature can be so widely accepted, while the other part, the Philosophy, or the Psychology, which deals with the inner nature of man, is so frequently neglected. We must remember the definition of this world of ours; it is only the Infinite Existence projected into the plane of consciousness. A little of the Infinite is projected into consciousness, and that we call our world. So there is an Infinite beyond, and religion has to deal with both, with the little lump we call our world, and with the Infinite beyond. Any religion which deals alone with either one of these two will be defective. It must deal with both. That part of religion which deals with this part of the Infinite which has come into this plane of consciousness, got itself caught, as it were, in the plane of consciousness, in the cage of time, space, and causation, is quite familiar to us, because we are in that already, and ideas about this world have been with us almost from time immemorial. The part of religion which deals with thc Infinite beyond comes entirely new to us, and getting ideas about it produces new channels in the brain, disturbing the whole system, and that is why you find in the practice of *Yoga* ordinary people are at first turned out of their groove. In order to lesson these disturbances as much as possible all these methods are devised by Patanjali, that we may practice any one of them best suited to us.

35

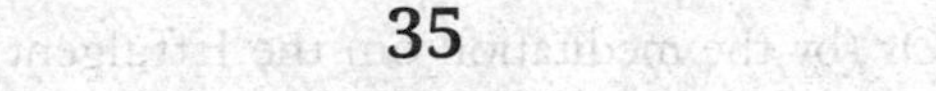

विषयवती वा प्रवृत्तिरुत्पन्ना मनसः स्थितिनिबन्धिनी

viṣayavatī vā pravṛtti-rutpannā manasaḥ sthiti-nibandhinī

> Those forms of concentration that bring extraordinary sense perceptions cause perseverance of the mind.

This naturally comes with *Dhāranā*, concentration; the *Yogis* say, if the mind becomes concentrated on the tip of the nose one begins to smell, after a few days, wonderful perfumes. If it becomes concentrated at the root of the tongue one begins to here sounds; if on the tip of the tongue one begins to taste wonderful flavours; if on the middle of the tongue, one feels as if he were coming in contact with something. If one concentrates his mind on the palate he begins to see peculiar things. If a man whose mind is disturbed wants to take up some of these practices of *Yoga*, yet doubts the truth of them, he will have his doubts set at rest, when, after a little practice, these things come to him, and he will persevere.

36

विशोका वा ज्योतिष्मती

viśokā vā jyotiṣmatī

> Or (by the meditation on) the Effulgent One which is beyond all sorrow.

This is another sort of concentration. Think of the lotus of the heart, with petals downwards, and running through it the *Sushumna*; take in the breath, and while throwing the breath out imagine that the lotus is turned with the petals upwards, and inside that lotus is an effulgent light. Meditate on that.

37

वीतरागविषयं वा चित्तम्

vītarāgaviṣayaṃ vā cittam

> Or (by meditation on) the heart that has given up all attachment to sense objects.

Take some holy person, some great person whom you revere, some saint whom you know to be perfectly non-attached, and think of his heart. That heart has become non-attached, and meditate on that heart; it will calm the mind. If you cannot do that, there is the next way.

38

स्वप्ननिद्राज्ञानालम्बनं वा

svapna-nidrā jñānālambanaṃ vā

Or by meditating on the knowledge that comes in sleep.

Sometimes a man dreams that he has seen angels coming to him and talking to him, that he is in an ecstatic condition, that he has heard music floating through the air. He is in a blissful condition in that dream, and when he awakes it makes a deep impression on him. Think of that dream as real, and meditate upon it. If you cannot do that, meditate on any holy thing that pleases you.

39

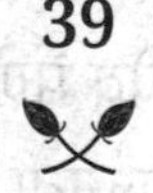

यथाभिमतध्यानाद्वा

yathābhimata-dhyānād-vā

Or by meditation on anything that appeals to one as good.

This does not mean any wicked subject, but anything good that you like, any place that you like best, any scenery that you like best, any idea that you like best, anything that will concentrate the mind.

40

परमाणुपरममहत्त्वान्तोऽस्य वशीकारः

paramāṇu-parama-mahattvānto'sya vaśīkāraḥ

The *Yogi*'s mind thus meditating, becomes unobstructed from the atomic to the Infinite.

The mind, by this practice, easily contemplates the most minute thing, as well as the biggest thing. Thus the mind waves become fainter.

41

क्षीणवृत्तेरभिजातस्येव मणेर्ग्रहीतृग्रहणग्राह्येषु
तत्स्थतद जनता समापत्ति

kṣīṇa-vṛtter-abhijātasyeva maṇer-grahītṛ-grahaṇa-grāhyeṣu tat-stha-tad-añjanatā samāpattiḥ

The *Yogi* whose *Vrttis* have thus become powerless (controlled) obtains in the receiver, receiving, and received (the self, the mind

> and external objects), concentratedness and sameness, like the crystal (before different coloured objects.)

What results from this constant meditation? We must remember how in a previous aphorism Patanjali went into the various states of meditation, and how the first will be the gross, and the second the fine objects, and from them the advance is to still finer objects of meditation, and how, in all these meditations, which are only of the first degree, not very high ones, we get as a result that we can meditate as easily on the fine as on the grosser objects. Here the *Yogi* sees the three things, the receiver, the received, and the receiving instrument, corresponding to the Soul, external objects, and the mind. There are three objects of meditation given to us. Firs the gross things, as bodies, or material objects, second fine things, as the mind, the *Chitta*, and third the *Purasa* qualified, not the *Purasa* itself, but the egoism. By practice, the *Yogi* gets established in all these meditations. Whenever he meditates he can keep out all other thought; he becomes identified with that on which he mediates; when he meditates he is like a piece of crystal; before flowers the crystal becomes almost identified with flowers. If the flower is red, the crystal looks red, or if the flower is blue, the crystal looks blue.

42

तत्र शब्दार्थज्ञानविकल्पैः संकीर्णा सवितर्का समापत्तिः

tatra śabdārtha-jñāna-vikalpaiḥ saṅkīrṇā savitarkā samāpattiḥ

> Sound, meaning, and resulting knowledge, being mixed up, is (called Samādhi) with reasoning.

Sound here means vibration; meaning, the nerve currents which conduct it; and knowledge, reaction. All the various meditations we have had so far, Patanjali calls *Savitarka* (meditations with reasoning). Later on he will give us higher and higher *Dhyānas.* In these that are called "with reasoning," we keep the duality of subject and object, which results from the mixture of word, meaning, and knowledge. There is first the external vibration, the word; this, carried inward by the sense currents, is the meaning. After that there comes a reactionary wave in the *Chitta*, which is knowledge, but the mixture of these three makeup what we call knowledge. In all the meditations up to this we get this mixture as object of meditation. The next *Samādhi* is higher.

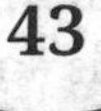

43

स्मृतिपरिशुद्धौ स्वरूपशून्येवार्थमात्रनिर्भासा निर्वितर्का

smṛti-pariśuddhau svarūpa-śūnyevārtha-mātra-nirbhāsā nirvitarkā

> The *Samādhi* called without reasoning (comes) when the memory is purified, or devoid of qualities, expressing only the meaning (of the meditated object).

It is by practice of meditation of these three that we come to the state where these three do not mix. We can get rid of them. We will first try to understand what these three are. Here is the *Chitta*; you will always remember the simile of the lake, the mind-stuff, and the vibration, the word, the sound, like a pulsation coming over it. You have that calm lake in you, and I pronounce a word, "cow." As soon as it enters through your ears there is a wave produced in your *Chitta* along with it. So that wave represents the idea of the cow, the form or the meaning as we call it. That apparent cow that you know is really that wave in the mind-stuff, and that comes as a reaction to the internal and external sound-vibrations, and with the sound, the wave dies away; that wave can never exist without a word. You may ask how it is when we only think of the cow, and do not hear a sound. You make that sound yourself. You are saying "cow" faintly in your mind, and with that comes a wave. There cannot be any wave without this impulse of sound, and when it is not from outside it is from inside, and when the sound dies, the wave dies. What remains? The result of the reaction, and that is knowledge. These three are so closely combined in our mind that we cannot separate them. When the sound comes, the senses vibrate, and the wave rises in reaction; they follow so closely upon one another that there is no discerning one from the other; when this meditation has been practiced for a long time, memory, the receptacle of all impressions, becomes purified, and we are able clearly to distinguish them from one another. This is called "*Nirvitarka*," concentration without reasoning.

44

एतयैव सविचारा निर्विचारा च सूक्ष्मविषया व्याख्याता

etayaiva savicārā nirvicārā ca sūkṣma-viṣaya vyākhyātā

> By this process (the concentrations) with discrimination and without discrimination, whose objects are finer, are (also) explained.

A process similar to the preceding is applied again, only, the objects to be taken up in the former meditations are gross; in this they are fine.

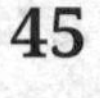

45

सूक्ष्मविषयत्वं चालिङ्गपर्यवसानम्

sūkṣma-viṣayatvaṃ cāliṅga-paryavasānam

The finer objects end with the *Pradhāna*.

The gross objects are only the elements, and everything manufactured out of them. The fine objects begin with the *Tanmātras* or fine particles. The organs, the mind*, egoism, the mind-stuff (the cause of all manifestion) the equilibrium state of *Sattva*, *Rajas* and *Tamas* materials—called *Pradhāna* (chief), *Prakrti* (nature), or *Avyakta* (unmanifest), are all included within the category of fine objects. The *Purusa* (the Soul) alone is excepted from this definition.

46

ता एव सबीजः समाधिः

tā eva sa-bījaḥ samādhiḥ

These concentrations are with seed.

These do not destroy the seeds of past actions, thus cannot give liberation, but what they bring to the *Yogi* is stated in the following aphorisms.

---

* The mind, or common sensory, the aggregate of all senses.

47

निर्विचारवैशारद्येऽध्यात्मप्रसादः

nirvicāra-vaiśāradye'dhyātma-prasādaḥ

The concentration "without reasoning" being purified, the Chitta becomes firmly fixed.

48

ऋतम्भरा तत्र प्रज्ञा

ṛtaṁbharā tatra prajñā

The knowledge in that is called "filled with Truth."

The next aphorism will explain this.

49

श्रुतानुमानप्रज्ञाभ्यामन्याविषया विशेषार्थत्वात्

śrutānumāna-prajñābhyām-anyaviṣayā viśeṣārthatvāt

The knowledge that is gained from testimony and inference is about common objects. That

> from the *Samādhi* just mentioned is of a much higher order, being able to penetrate where inference and testimony cannot go.

The idea is that we have to get our knowledge of ordinary objects by direct perception, and by inference therefrom, and from testimony of people who are competent. By "people who are competent," the *Yogis* always mean the *Rishis*, or the Seers of the thoughts recorded in the Scriptures—the *Vedas*. According to them, the only proof of the Scriptures is that they were the testimony of competent persons, yet they say the Scriptures cannot take us to realisation. We can read all the *Vedas*, and yet will not realise anything, but when we practise their teachings, then we attain to that state which realises what the Scriptures say, which penetrates where reason cannot go, and where the testimony of others cannot avail. This is what is meant by this aphorism, that realisation is real religion, and all the rest is only preparation—hearing lectures, or reading books, or reasoning, is merely preparing the ground; it is not religion. Intellectual assent, and intellectual dissent are not religion. The central idea of the *Yogis* is that just as we come in direct contact with the objects of the senses, so religion can be directly perceived in a far more intense sense. The truths of religion, as God and Soul, cannot be perceived by the external senses. I cannot see God with my eyes, nor can I touch Him with my hands, and we also know that neither can we reason beyond the senses. Reason leaves us at a point quite indecisive; we may reason all our lives, as the world has been doing for thousands of years, and the result is that we find we are incompetent to prove or disprove the facts of religion. What we perceive directly we take as the basis, and upon that basis we reason. So it is obvious that reasoning has to run within these bounds of perception. It can never go beyond: the whole scope of realisation, therefore, is beyond sense perception. The *Yogis* say that man can go beyond his direct sense perception, and beyond his reason also. Man has in him the faculty, the power, of transcending his intellect even, and that power is in every being, every creature. By the practice of *Yoga* that power is aroused, and then man transcends the ordinary limits of reason, and directly perceives things which are beyond all reason.

50

तज्जः संस्कारोऽन्यसंस्कारप्रतिबन्धी

taj-jaḥ saṃskāro'nya-saṃskāra-pratibandhī

> The resulting impression from this *Samādhi* obstructs all other impressions.

We have seen in the foregoing aphorism that the only way of attaining to that superconsciousness is by concentration, and we have also seen that what hinder the mind from concentration are the past *Samskāras*, impressions. All of you have observed that when you are trying to concentrate your mind, your thoughts wander. When you are trying to think of God, that is the very time which all these *Samskāras* take to appear. At other times they are not so active, but when you want them not to be they are sure to be there, trying their best to crowd inside your mind. Why should that be so? Why should they be much more potent at the time of concentration? It is because you are repressing them and they react with all their force. At other times they do not react. How countless these old past impressions must be, all lodge somewhere in the *Chitta*, ready, waiting like tigers to jump up. These have to be suppressed that the one idea which we like may arise, to the exclusion of the others. Instead, they are all struggling to come up at the same time. These are the various powers of the *Samskāras* in hindering concentration of the mind, so this *Samādhi* which has just been given is the best to be practised, on account of its power of suppressing the *Samskāras*. The *Samskāra* which will be raised by this sort of concentration will be so powerful that it will hinder the action of the others, and hold them in check.

51

तस्यापि निरोधे सर्वनिरोधान्निर्बीजः समाधिः

tasyāpi nirodhe sarva-nirodhān-nirbījaḥ samādhiḥ

> By the restraint of even this (impression, which obstructs all other impressions), all being restrained, comes the "seedless" *Samādhi.*

You remember that our goal is to perceive the Soul itself. We cannot perceive the Soul because it has got mingled up with nature, with the mind, with the body. The most ignorant man thinks his body is the Soul. The more learned man thinks his mind is the Soul, but both of these are mistaken. What makes the Soul get mingled up with all this, these different waves in the *Chitta* rise and cover the Soul, and we only are a little reflection of the Soul through these waves, so, if the wave be one of anger, we see the Soul as angry: "I am angry," we say. If the wave is a wave of love we see ourselves reflected in that wave, and say we are loving. If that wave is one of weakness, and the Soul is reflected in it, we think we are weak. Thcsc various idcas comc from thcsc imprcssions, thcse *Samskāras* covering the Soul. The real nature of the Soul is not perceived until all the waves have subsided; so, first, Patanjali teaches us the meaning of these waves; secondly, the best way to repress them; and thirdly, how to make one wave so strong as to suppress all other waves, fire eating fire as it were. When only one remains, it will be easy to suppress that also, and when that is gone, this *Samādhi* of concentration is called seedless; it leaves nothing, and the Soul is manifested just as It is, in Its own glory. Then alone we know that the Soul is not a compound, It is the only eternal simple in the universe, and, as such, It cannot be born, It cannot die, It is immortal, indestructible, the ever-living essence of intelligence.

PART II

SADHANA PADA

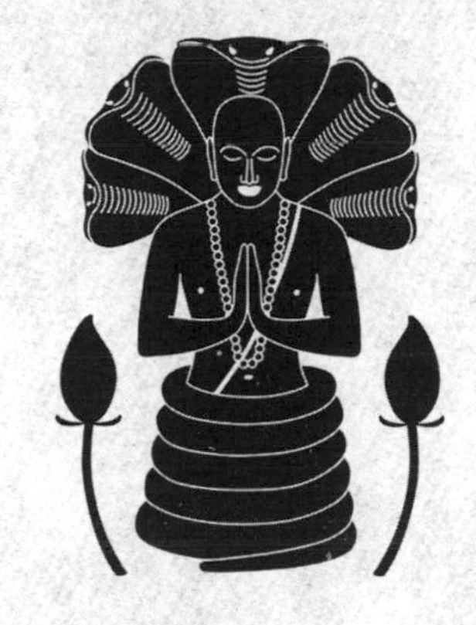

Concentration – Its Practice

॥ द्वितीयः साधनपादः ॥

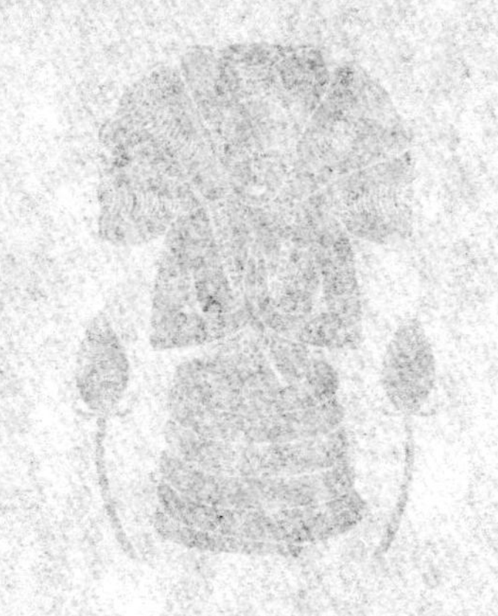

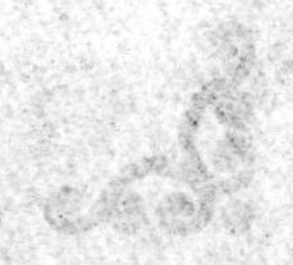

1

तपः स्वाध्यायेश्वरप्रणिधानानि क्रियायोगः

tapaḥ svādhyāyeśvarapraṇidhānāni kriyā-yogaḥ

Mortification, study, and surrendering fruits of work to God are called *Kriyā Yoga.*

Those *Samādhis* with which we ended our last chapter are very difficult to attain; so we must take them up slowly. The first step, the preliminary step, is called *Kriyā Yoga.* Literally this means work, working towards *Yoga.* The organs are the horses, the mind is the reins, the intellect is the charioteer, the soul is the rider, and this body is the chariot. The master of the household, the King, the Self of man, is sitting in this chariot. If the horses are very strong, and do not obey the reins, if the charioteer, the intellect, does not know how to control the horses, then this chariot will come to grief. But if the organs, the horses, are well controlled, and if the reins, the mind, are well held in the hands of the charioteer, the intellect, the chariot, reaches the goal. What is meant, therefore, by mortification? Holding the reins firmly while guiding this body and mind: not letting the body do anything it likes, but keeping them both in proper control. *Study*. What is meant by study in this case? Not study of novels, or fiction, or story books, but study of those books which teach the liberation of the soul. Then again this study does not mean controversial studies at all. The *Yogi* is supposed to have finished his period of controversy. He has had enough of all that, and has become satisfied. He only studies to intensify his convictions. *Vadā* and *Siddhānta*. These are the two sorts of Scriptural knowledge, *Vadā* (the argumentative) and *Siddhānta* (the decisive). When a man is entirely ignorant he takes up the first part of this, the argumentative fighting, and reasoning, pros and cons; and when he has finished that he takes up the *Siddhānta*, the decisive, arriving at a conclusion. Simply arriving at this conclusion will not do. It must be intensified. Books are infinite in number, and time is short; therefore this is the secret of knowledge, to take that which is essential. Take that out, and then try to live up to it. There is an old simile in India that if you place a cup of milk before a *Rāja Hamsa* (swan) with plenty of water in it, he will take all the milk and leave the water. In that way we should take what is of value in knowledge, and leave the dross. All these intellectual gymnastics are necessary at first. We must not go blindly into anything. The *Yogi* has passed the argumentative stage, and has come to a conclusion, which is like the rocks, immovable. The only thing he now seeks to do is intensify that conclusion. Do not argue, he says; if one forces arguments upon you, be silent. Do not answer any argument, but go away free, because arguments only disturb the mind. The only thing is to train the intellect, so what is the use of disturbing it any more. The intellect is but a weak instrument, and can give only knowledge limited by the senses; the *Yogi* wants to go beyond the senses; therefore the intellect is of no use to him. He is certain of this, and therefore is silent, and does not argue. Every argument throws his mind out of balance, creates a disturbance in the *Chitta*, and this disturbance is a drawback. These argumentations and searchings of the reason are only on the way. There are much higher things behind them. The whole of life is not for schoolboy fights and debating societies. By "surrendering the fruits of work to God" is to take to ourselves neither credit nor blame, but to give both up to the Lord, and be at peace.

2

समाधिभावनार्थः क्लेशतनूकरणार्थश्च

samādhi-bhāvanārthaḥ kleśa-tanū-karaṇārthaś ca

(They are for) the practice of *Samādhi* and minimising the pain-bearing obstructions.

Most of us make our minds like spoiled children, allowing them to do whatever they want. Therefore it is necessary that there should be constant practice of the previous mortifications, in order to gain control of the mind, and bring it into subjection. The obstructions to *Yoga* arise from lack of this control, and cause us pain. They can only be removed by denying the mind, and holding it in check, through these various means.

3

अविद्यास्मितारागद्वेषाभिनिवेशाः क्लेशाः

avidyāsmitā-rāga-dveṣābhiniveśāḥ kleśāḥ

> The pain-bearing obstructions are—ignorance, egoism, attachment, aversion, and clinging to life.

These are the five pains, the fivefold tie that binds us down. Of course ignorance is the mother of all the rest. She is the only cause of all our misery. What else can make us miserable? The nature of the Soul is eternal bliss. What can make it sorrowful except ignorance, hallucination, delusion; all this pain of the soul is simply delusion.

4

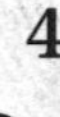

अविद्या क्षेत्रमुत्तरेषां प्रसुप्ततनुविच्छिन्नोदाराणाम्

avidyā kṣetram-uttareṣām prasupta-tanuvicchinnodārāṇām

> Ignorance is the productive field of all them that follow, whether they are dormant, attenuated, overpowered, or expanded.

Impressions are the cause of these, and these impressions exist in different degrees. There are the dormant. You often hear the expression "innocent as a baby," yet in the baby may be the state of a demon or of a god which will come out by and by. In the *Yogi* these impressions, the *Samskāras* left by past actions, are attenuated; that is, in a very fine state, and he can control them, and not allow them to become manifest. Overpowered means that sometimes one set of impressions is held down for a while by those that are stronger, but they will come out when that repressing cause is removed. The last state is the expanded, when the *Samskāras*, having helpful surroundings, have attained to great activity, either as good or evil.

5

अनित्याशुचिदुःखानात्मसु नित्यशुचिसुखात्मख्यातिरविद्या

anityāśuci-duḥkhānātmasu nitya-śuci-sukhātma-khyātir-avidyā

> Ignorance is taking that which is non-eternal, impure, painful, and non-Self, for the eternal, pure, happy, Atmān (Self).

All these various sorts of impression have one source: ignorance. We have first to learn what ignorance is. All of us think that "I am the body," and not the Self, the pure, the effulgent, the ever blissful, and that is ignorance. We think of man, and see man as body. This is the great delusion.

6

दृग्दर्शनशक्त्योरेकात्मतेवास्मिता

dṛg-darśana-śaktyor-ekātmata-ivāsmitā

Egoism is the identification of the seer with the instrument of seeing.

The seer is really the Self, the pure one, the ever holy, the infinite, the immortal. That is the Self of man. And what are the instruments? The *Chitta*, or mind-stuff, the *Buddhi*, determinative faculty, the *Manas*, or mind, and the *Indriyani*, or sense organs. These are the instruments for him to see the external world, and the identification of the Self with the instruments is what is called the ignorance of egoism. We say "I am the mind, I am thought; I am angry, or I am happy." How can we be angry, and how can we hate? We should identify ourselves with the Self; that cannot change. If it is unchangeable, how can it be one moment happy, and one moment unhappy? It is formless, infinite, omnipresent. What can change it? Beyond all law. What can affect it? Nothing in the universe can produce an effect on it, yet, through ignorance, we identify ourselves with the mind-stuff, and think we feel pleasure or pain.

7

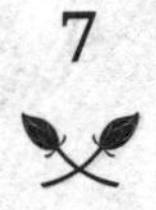

सुखानुशयी रागः

sukhānuśayī rāgaḥ

Attachment is that which dwells on pleasure.

We find pleasure in certain things, and the mind, like a current, flows towards them, and that, following the pleasure centre, as it were, is attachment. We are never attached to anyone in whom we do not find pleasurc. Wc find pleasure in very queer things sometimes, but the definition is just the same; wherever we find pleasure, there we are attached.

8

दुःखानुशयी द्वेषः

duḥkhānuśayī dveṣaḥ

Aversion is that which dwells on pain.

That, which gives us pain we immediately seek to get away from.

9

स्वरसवाही विदुषोऽपि तथारूढोऽभिनिवेशः

sva-rasvāhi viduṣo'pi samārūḍho'bhiniveśaḥ

> Flowing through its own nature, and established even in the learned, is the clinging to life.

This clinging to life you see manifested in every animal, and upon it many attempts have been made to build the theory of a future life, because men like their lives so much that they desire a future life also. Of course it goes without saying that this argument is without much value, but the most curious part of it is that, in Western Countries, the idea that this clinging to life indicates a possibility of a future life applies only to men, but does not include animals. In India this clinging to life has been one of the arguments to prove past experience and existence. For instance, if it be true that all our knowledge has come from experience, then it is sure that that which we never experienced we cannot imagine, or understand. As soon as chickens are hatched they begin to pick up food. Many times it has been seen where ducks have been hatched by hens, that, as soon as they come out of the eggs, they flew to water, and the mother thought they would be drowned. If experience be the only source of knowledge, where did these chickens learn to pick up food, or the ducklings that the water was their natural element? If you say it is instinct, it means nothing—it is simply giving it a word, but is no explanation. What is this instinct? We have many instincts in ourselves. For instance, most of you ladies play the piano, and remember, when you first learned, how carefully you had to put your fingers on the black and the white keys, one after the other, but now, after long years of practice, you can talk with your friends, and your hand goes on just the same. It has become instinct, it becomes automatic, but so far as we know, all the cases which we now regard as automatic are degenerated reason. In the language of the *Yogi*, instinct is involved reason. Discrimination becomes involved, and gets to be automatic *Samskāras*. Therefore it is perfectly logical to think that all we call instinct in this world is simply involved reason. As reason cannot come without experience, all instinct is, therefore, the result of past experience. Chickens fear the hawk, and ducklings love the water, and these are both the result of past experience, and these are both the result of past experience. Then the question is whether that experience belongs to a particular soul, or to the body simply, whether this experience which comes to the duck is the duck's forefather's experience, or the duck's own experience. Modern scientific men hold that it belongs to the body, but the *Yogis* hold that it is the experience of the soul, transmitted through the body. This is called the theory of reincarnation. We have seen that all of our knowledge, whether we call it perception or reason, or instinct, must come through that one channel called experience, and all that we know call instinct is the result of past experience, degenerated into instinct, and that instinct regenerates into reason again. So on throughout the universe, and upon this has been built one of the chief arguments for reincarnation, in India.

The recurring experiences of various fears, in course of time, produce this clinging to life. That is why the child is instinctively afraid, because the past experience of pain is there. Even in the most learned men, who know that this body will go, and who say "never mind: we have hundreds of bodies; the soul cannot die"—even in them, with all their intellectual conviction, we still find this clinging to life. What is this clinging to life? We have seen that it has become instinctive. In the psychological language of *Yoga* if has become *Samskāras*. The *Samskāras*, fine and hidden, are sleeping in the *Chitta*. All these past experiences of death, all that which we call instinct, is experience become sub-conscious. It lives in the *Chitta*, and is not inactive, but is working underneath. These *Chitta Vrttis*, these mind-waves, which are gross, we can appreciate and feel; they can be more easily controlled, but what about these finer instincts? How can they be controlled? When I am angry my whole mind has become a huge wave of anger. Feel it, see it, handle it, can easily manipulate it, can fight with it, but I shall not succeed perfectly in the fight until I can get down below. A man says something very harsh to me, and I begin to feel that I am getting heated, and he goes on until I am perfectly angry, and forget myself, identify myself with anger. When he first began to abuse me I still thought "I am going to be angry." Anger was one thing and I was another, but when I became angry, I was anger. These feelings have to be controlled in the germ, the root, in their fine forms, before even we have become conscious that they are acting on us. With the vast majority of mankind the fine states of these passions are not even known, the state when they are slowly coming from beneath consciousness. When a bubble is rising from the bottom of the lake we do not see it, or even when it is nearly come to the surface; it is only when it bursts and makes a ripple that we know it is there. We shall only be successful in grappling with the waves when we can get hold of them in their fine causes, and until you can get hold of them, and subdue them before any become gross, there is no hope of conquering any passion perfectly. To control our passions we have to control them at their very roots; then alone shall we be able to burn out their very seed. As fried seeds thrown into the ground will never come up, so these passions will never arise.

10

ते प्रतिप्रसवहेयाः सूक्ष्माः

te pratiprasava-heyāḥ sūkṣmāḥ

> They, to-be-rejected-by-opposite-modifications, are fine.

How are these fine *Samskāras* to be controlled? We have to begin with the big waves, and come down and down. For instance, when a big wave of anger has come into the mind, how are we to control that? Just by raising a big opposing wave. Think of love. Sometimes a mother is very angry with her husband, and while in that state the baby comes in, and she kisses the baby; the old wave dies out, and a new wave arises, love for the child. That suppresses the other one. Love is opposite to anger. So we find that by raising the opposite waves we can conquer those which we want to reject. Then, if we can raise in our fine nature those fine opposing waves, they will check the fine workings of anger beneath the conscious surface. We have seen now that all these instinctive actions first began as conscious actions, and became finer and finer. So, if good waves in the conscious *Chitta* be constantly raised, they will go down, become subtle, and oppose the *Samskāra* forms of evil thoughts.

11

ध्यानहेयास्तद्वृत्तयः

dhyāna-heyās-tad-vṛttayaḥ

> By meditation, their modifications are to be rejected.

Meditation is one of the great means of controlling the rising of these big waves. By meditation you can make the mind subdue these waves, and, if you go on practising meditation for days, and months, and years, until it has become a habit, until it will come in spite of yourself, anger and hatred will be controlled and checked.

12

क्लेशमूलः कर्माशयो दृष्टादृष्टजन्मवेदनीयः

kleśa-mūlaḥ karmāśayo dṛṣṭādṛṣṭa-janma-vedanīyaḥ

> The receptacle of works has its root in these pain-bearing obstructions, and their experience in this visible life, or in the unseen life.

By the receptacle of works is meant the sum-total of these *Samskāras*. Whatever work we do, the mind is thrown into a wave, and, after the work is finished, we think the wave is gone. No. It has only become fine, but it is still there. When we try to remember the thing, it comes up again and becomes a wave. So it was there; if it had not been there, there would not have been memory. So, every action, every thought, good or bad, just goes down and becomes fine, and is there stored up. They are called pain-bearing obstructions, both happy and unhappy thoughts, because according to the *Yogis*, both, in the long run, bring pain. All happiness which comes from the senses will, eventually, bring pain. All enjoyment will make us thirst for more, and that brings pain as its result. There is no limit to man's desires; he goes on desiring, and when he comes to a point where desire cannot be fulfilled, the result is pain. Therefore the *Yogis* regard the sum-total of the impressions, good or evil, as pain-bearing obstructions; they obstruct the way to freedom of the Soul. It is the same with the *Samskāras*, the fine roots of all our works: they are the causes which will again bring effects, either in this life, or in the lives to come. In exceptional cases, when these *Samskāras* are very strong, they bear fruit quickly; exceptional acts of wickedness, or of goodness, bring their fruits in this life. The *Yogis* even hold that men who are able to acquire a tremendous power of good *Samskāras* do not have to die, but, even in this life, can change their bodies into god-bodies. There are several cases mentioned by the *Yogis* in their books. These men change the very material of their bodies; they rearrange the molecules in such fashion that they have no more sickness, and what we call death does not come to them. Why should not this be? The physiological meaning of foot is assimilation of energy from the sun. This energy has reached the plant, the plant is eaten by an animal, and the animal by us. The science of it is that we take so much energy from the sun, and make it part of ourselves. That being the case, why should there be only one way of assimilating energy? The plant's way is not the same as ours; the earth's process of assimilating energy differs from our own. But all assimilate energy in some form or other. The *Yogis* say that they are able to assimilate energy by the power of the mind alone, that they can draw in as much as they desire without recourse to the ordinary methods. As a spider makes his net out of his own substance, and becomes bound in his net, and cannot go anywhere except along the lines of that net, so we have projected out of our own substance this network called the nerves, and we cannot work except through the channels of those nerves. The *Yogi* says we need not be bound by that. Similarly, we can send electricity to any part of the world, but we have to send it by means of wires. Nature can send a vast mass of electricity without any wires at all. Why cannot we do the same? We can send mental electricity. What we call mind is very much the same as electricity. It is clear that this nerve fluid has some amount of electricity, because it is polarised, and it answers all electrical directions. We can only send our electricity through these nerve channels. Why not send the mental electricity without this aid? The *Yogi* says it is perfectly possible and practicable, and that when you can do that you will work all over the universe. You will be able to work with anybody anywhere, without the help of any nervous system. When the soul is acting through these channels we say a man is living and when those channels die the man is said to be said. But when a man is able to act either with or without these channels, birth and death will have no meaning for him. All the bodies in the universe are made up of *Tanmātras*, and it is only in the arrangement of them that there comes a difference. If you are the arranger you can arrange that body in one way or another. Who makes up this body but you? Who eats the food? If another ate the food for you, you would not live long. Who makes the blood out of it? You, certainly. Who assimilates the blood, and sends it through the veins? You. Who creates the nerves, and makes all the muscles? You are the manufacturer, out of your own substance. You are the manufacturer of the body, and you live in it. Only we have lost the knowledge of how to make it. We have become automatic, degenerate. We have forgotten the process of manufacture. So, what we do automatically has again to be regulated. We are the creators and we have to regulate that creation, and as soon as we can do that we shall be able to manufacture just as we like, and then we shall have neither birth nor death, disease, or anything.

13

सति मूले तद्विपाको जात्यायुर्भोगाः

sati mūle tad-vipāko jātyāyur-bhogāḥ

The root being there, the fruition comes (in the form of) species, life, and expression of pleasure and pain.

The roots, the causes, the *Samskāras* being there, they again manifest, and form the effects. The cause dying down becomes the effect, and the effect becomes more subtle, and becomes the cause of the next effect. The tree bears a seed, and becomes the cause of the next tree, and so on. All our works now, are the effects of past *Samskāras*. Again, these *Samskāras* become the cause of future actions, and thus we go on. So this aphorism says that the cause being there, the fruit must come, in the form of species; one will be a man, another an angel, another an animal, another a demon. Then there are different effects in life; one man lives fifty years, another a hundred, and another dies in two years, and never attains maturity; all these differences in life are regulated by these past actions. One man is born, as it were, for pleasure; if he buries himself in a forest pleasure will follow him there. Another man, wherever he goes, pain follows him, everything becomes painful. It is all the result of their own past. According to the philosophy of the *Yogis* all virtuous actions bring pleasure, and all vicious actions bring pain. Any man who does wicked deeds is sure to reap the fruit of them in the form of pain.

14

ते ह्लादपरितापफलाः पुण्यापुण्यहेतुत्वात्

te hlāda-paritāpa-phalāḥ puṇyāpuṇya-hetutvāt

They bear fruit as pleasure or pain, caused by virtue or vice.

15

परिणामतापसंस्कारदुःखैर्गुणवृत्तिविरोधाच्च
दुःखमेव सर्वं विवेकिनः

pariṇāma-tāpa-saṃskāra-duḥkhaiḥ guṇa-vṛtti-virodhācca duḥkham-eva sarvaṃ vivekinaḥ

> To the discriminating, all is, as it were, painful on account of everything bringing pain, either in the consequences, or in apprehension, or in attitude caused by impressions, also on account of the counteraction of qualities.

The *Yogis* say that the man who has discriminating powers, the man of good sense, sees through all these various things, which are called pleasure and pain, and knows that they are always equally distributed, and that one follows the other, and melts into the other; he sees that men are following an *ignis fatuus* all their lives, and never succeed in fulfilling their desires. There was never a love in this world which did not know decay. The great king *Yudisthira* once said that the most wonderful thing in life is that every moment we see people dying around us, and yet we think we shall never die. Surrounded by fools on every side, we think we are the only exceptions, the only learned men. Surrounded by all sorts of experiences of fickleness, we think our love is the only lasting love. How can that be? Even love is selfish, and the *Yogi* says that, in the end, we shall find that even the love of husbands and wives, and children and friends, slowly decays. Decadence seizes everything in this life. It is only when everything, even love, fails, that, with a flash, man finds out how vain, how dream-like is this world. Then he catches a glimpse of *Vairāgyam* (renunciation), catches a glimpse of the beyond. It is only by giving up this world that the other comes; never through building on to this one. Never yet was there a great soul who had not to reject sense pleasures and enjoyments to become such. The cause of misery is the clash between difference forces of nature, one dragging one way, and another dragging another, rendering permanent happiness impossible.

16

हेयं दुःखमनागतम्

heyaṃ duḥkham-anāgatam

> The misery which is not yet come is to be avoided.

Some *Karma* we have worked out already, some we are working out now in the present, and some is waiting to bear fruit in the future. That which we have worked out already is past and gone.

That which we are experiencing now we will have to work out, and it is only that which is waiting to bear fruit in the future that we can conquer and control, so all our forces should be directed towards the control of that *Karma* which has not yet borne fruit. That is meant in the previous aphorism, when Patanjali says that these various *Samskāras* are to be controlled by counteracting waves.

17

द्रष्टृदृश्ययोः संयोगो हेयहेतुः

draṣṭṛ -dṛśyayoḥ saṃyogo heya-hetuḥ

The cause of that which is to be avoided is the junction of the seer and the seen.

Who is the seer? The Self of Man, the *Purusa*. What is the seen? The whole of nature, beginning with the mind, down to gross matter. All this pleasure and pain arises from the junction between this *Purusa* and the mind. The *Purusa*, you must remember, according to this philosophy, is pure; it is when it is joined to nature, and by reflection, that it appears to feel either pleasure or pain.

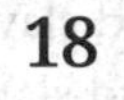

18

प्रकाशक्रियास्थितिशीलं भूतेन्द्रियात्मकं भोगापवर्गार्थं दृश्यम्

prakāśa-kriyā-sthiti-śīlaṃ bhūtendriyātmakaṃ bhogāpavargārthaṃ dṛśyam

The experienced is composed of elements and organs, is of the nature of illumination, action and inertia, and is for the purpose of experience and release (of the experiencer).

The experienced, that is nature, is composed of elements and organs—the elements gross and fine which compose the whole of nature, and the organs of the senses, mind, etc., and is of the nature of illumination, action, and inertia. These are what in Sanskrit are called *Sattva* (illumination), *Rajas* (action), and *Tamas* (darkness); each is for the purpose of experience and release. What is the purpose of the whole of nature? That the *Purusa* may gain experience. The *Purusa* has, as it were, forgotten its mighty, godly, nature. There is a story that the king of the gods, *Indra*, once became a pig, wallowing in mire; he had a she pig, and a lot of baby pigs, and was very happy. Then some other angels saw his plight, and came to him, and told him, "You are the king of the gods, you have all the gods command. Why are you here?" But *Indra* said, "Let me be; I am all right here; I do not care for the heavens, while I have this sow and these little pigs." The poor gods were at their wits' end what to do. After a time they decided to slowly come and slay one of the little pigs, and then another, until they had slain all the pigs, and the sow too. When all were dead *Indra* began to weep and mourn. Then the gods ripped his pig-body open and he came out of it, and began to laugh when he realised what a hideous dream he had had—he, the king of the gods, to have become a pig, and to think that the pig-life was the only life! Not only so, but to have wanted the whole universe to come into the pig-life! The *Purusa*, when it identifies itself with nature, forgets that it is pure and infinite. The *Purusa* does not live; it is life itself. It does not exist; it is existence itself. The Soul does not know; it is knowledge itself. It is an entire mistake to say that the Soul lives, or knows, or loves. Love and existence are not the qualities of the *Purusa*, but its essence. When they get reflected upon something you may call them the qualities of that something. But they are not the qualities of the *Purusa*, but the essence of this great *Atmān*, this Infinite Being, without birth or death, Who is established in His own glory, but appears as if become degenerate until if you approach to tell Him, "You are not a pig," he begins to squeal and bite. Thus with us all in this *Māyā*, this dream world, where it is all misery, weeping, and crying, where a few golden balls are rolled, and the world scrambles after them. You were never bound by laws, Nature never had a bond for you. That is what the *Yogi* tells you; have patience to learn it. And the *Yogi* shows how, by junction with this nature, and identifying itself with the mind and the world, the *Purusa* thinks itself miserable. Then the *Yogi* goes on to show that the way out is through experience. You have to get all this experience, but finish it quickly. We have placed ourselves in this net, and will have to get out. We have got ourselves caught in the trap, and we will have to work out our freedom. So get this experience of husbands and wives, and friends, and little loves, and you will get through them safely if you never forget what you really are. Never forget this is only a momentary state, and that we have to pass through it. Experience is the one great teacher—experiences of pleasure and pain—but know they are only experiences, and will all lead, step by step, to that state when all these things will become small, and the *Purusa* will be so great that this whole universe will be as a drop in the ocean, and will fall off by its own nothingness. We have to go through these experiences, but let us never forget the ideal.

19

विशेषाविशेषलिङ्गमात्रालिङ्गानि गुणपर्वाणि

viśeṣāviśeṣa-liṅgamātrāliṅgāni guṇa-parvāṇi

The states of the qualities are the defined, the undefined, the indicated only, and the signless.

The system of *Yoga* is built entirely on the philosophy of the *Sānkhyas*, as I told you in some of the previous lectures, and here again I will remind you of the cosmology of the *Sānkhya* philosophy. According to the *Sānkhyas*, nature is both the material and efficient cause of this universe. In this nature there are three sorts of materials, the *Sattva*, the *Rajas*, and the *Tamas*. The *Tamas* material is all that is dark, all that is ignorant and heavy; and the *Rajas* is activity. The *Sattvas* is calmness, light. When nature is in the state before creation, it is called by them *Avyakta*, undefined, or indiscrete; that is, in which there is no distinction of form or name, a state in which these three materials are held in perfect balance. Then the balance is disturbed, these different materials begin to mingle in various fashions, and the result is this universe. In every man, also, these three materials exist. When the *Sattva* material prevails knowledge comes. When the *Rajas* material prevails activity comes, and when the *Tamas* material prevails darkness comes and lassitude, idleness, ignorance. According to the *Sānkhya* theory, the highest manifestation of this nature, consisting of these three materials, is what they call *Mahat*, or intelligence, universal intelligence, and each human mind is a part of that cosmic intelligence. Then out of *Mahat* comes the mind. In the *Sāṅkhya* Psychology there is a sharp distinction between *Manas*, the mind function, and the function of the *Buddhi* intellect. The mind function is simply to collect and carry impressions and present them to the *Buddhi*, the individual *Mahat*, and the *Buddhi* determined upon it. So, out of *Mahat* comes mind, and out of mind comes fine material, and this fine material combines and becomes the gross material outside—the external universe. The claim of the *Sāṅkhya* philosophy is that beginning with the intellect, and coming down to a block of stone, all has come out of the same thing, only as finer or grosser states of existence. The *Buddhi* is the finest state of existence of the materials, and then comes *Ahamkara*, egoism, and next to the mind comes fine material, which they call *Tanmātras*, which cannot be seen, but which are inferred. These *Tanmātras* combine and become grosser, and finally produce this universe. The finer is the cause, and the grosser is the effect. It begins with the *Buddhi*, which is the finest material, and goes on becoming grosser and grosser, until it becomes this universe. According to the *Sāṅkhya* philosophy, beyond the whole of this nature is the *Purusa*, which is not material at all. *Purusa* is not at all similar to anything else, either *Buddhi*, or mind, or the *Tanmātras*, or the gross material; it is not akin to any one of these, it is entirely separate, entirely different in its nature, and from this they argue that the *Purusa* must be immortal, because it is not the result of combination. That which is not the result of combination cannot die, these *Purusas* or Souls are infinite in number. Now we shall understand the Aphorism, that the states of the qualities are defined, undefined, and signless. By the defined is meant the gross elements, which we can sense. By the undefined is meant the very fine materials, the *Tanmātras*, which cannot be sensed by ordinary men. If you practice *Yoga*, however, says Patanjali, after a while your perception will become so fine that you will actually see the *Tanmātras*. For instance, you have heard how every man has a certain light about him; every living being is emanating a certain light, and this, he says, can be seen by the *Yogi*. We do not all see it, but we are all throwing out these *Tanmātras*, just as a flower is continuously emanating these *Tanmātras*, which enable us to smell it. Every day of our lives we are throwing out a mass of good or evil, and everywhere we go the atmosphere is full of these materials, and that is how there came to the human mind, even unconsciously, the idea of building temples and churches? Why should man build churches in which to worship God? Why not worship Him anywhere? Even if he did not know the reason, man found that that place where people worshipped God became full of good *Tanmātras*. Every day people go there, and the more they go the holier they get, and the holier that place becomes. If any man who has not much *Sattva* in him goes there the place will influence him, and arouse his *Sattva* quality. Here, therefore, is the significance of all temples and holy places, but you must remember that their holiness depends on holy people congregating there. The difficulty with mankind is that they forget the original meaning, and put the cart before the horse. It was men who made these places holy, and then the effect became the cause and made men holy. If the wicked only were to go there it would become as bad as any other place. It is not the building, but the people, that make a church, and that is what we always forget. That is why sages and holy persons, who have so much of this *Sattva* quality, are emanating so much of it around them, and exerting a tremendous influence day and night on their surroundings. A man may become so pure that his purity will become tangible, as it were. The body has become pure, and in an intensely physical sense, no figurative idea, no poetical language, it emanates that purity wherever it goes. Whosoever comes in contact with that man becomes pure. Next "the indicated only" means the *Buddhi*, the intellect. "The indicated only" is the first manifestation of nature; from it all other manifestations proceed. The last is "the signless." Here there seems to be a great fight between modern science and all religion. Every religion has this idea that this universe comes out of intelligence. Only some religions were more philosophical, and used scientific language. The very theory of God, taking it in its psychological significance, and apart from all ideas of personal God, is that intelligence is first in the order of creation, and that out of intelligence comes what we call gross matter. Modern philosophers say that intelligence is the last to come. They say that unintelligent things slowly evolve into animals, and from animals slowly evolve into men. They claim that instead of everything coming out of intelligence, intelligence is itself the last to come. Both the religious and the scientific statement, though seemingly directly opposed to each other, are true. Take an infinite series A—B—A—B—A—B, etc. The question is which is first, A or B. If you take the series as A—, you will say that A is first, but if you take it as B—A you will say that B is first. It depends on the way you are looking at it. Intelligence evolves, and becomes the gross material, and this again evolves as intelligence, and again evolves as matter once more. The *Sānkhyas*, and all religionists, put intelligence first, and the series becomes intelligence then matter, intelligence then matter. The scientific man puts his finger on matter, and say matter then intelligence, matter then intelligence. But they are both indicating the same chain. Indian philosophy, however, goes beyond both intelligence and matter, and finds a *Purusa*, or Self, which is beyond all intelligence, and of which intelligence is but the borrowed light.

20

द्रष्टादृशिमात्रः शुद्धोऽपि प्रत्ययानुपश्यः

draṣṭā-dṛśi-mātraḥ śuddho'pi pratyayānupaśyaḥ

> The seer is intelligence only, and though pure,
> seen through the colouring of the intellect.

This is again *Sānkhya* philosophy. We have seen from this philosophy that from the lowest form up to intelligence all is nature, but beyond nature are *Purusas* (souls), and these have no qualities. Then how does the soul appear to be happy or unhappy? By reflection. Just as if be piece of pure crystal be put on a table and a red flower be put near it, the crystal appears to be red, so all these appearances of happiness or unhappiness are but reflections; the soul itself has no sort of colouring. The soul is separate from nature; nature is one thing, soul another, eternally separate. The *Sānkhyas* say that intelligence is a compound, that it grows and wanes, that it changes, just as the body changes, and that its nature is nearly the same as that of the body. As a fingernail is to the body, so is body to intelligence. The nail is a part of the body, but it can be pared off hundreds of times, and the body will still last. Similarly, the intelligence lasts æons, while this body can be pared off, thrown off. Yet intelligence cannot be immortal, because it changes—growing and waning. Anything that changes cannot be immortal. Certainly intelligence is manufactured, and that very fact shows us that there must be something beyond that, because it cannot be free. Everything connected with matter is in nature, and therefore bound for ever. Who is free? That free one must certainly be beyond cause and effect. If you say that the idea of freedom is a delusion, I will say that the idea of bondage is also a delusion. Two facts come into our consciousness, and stand or fall by each other. One is that we are bound. If we want to go through a wall, and our head bumps against that wall, we are limited by that wall. At the same time we find will, and think we can direct our will everywhere. At every step these contradictory ideas are coming to us. We have to believe that we are free, yet at every moment we find we are not free. If one idea is a delusion, the other is also a delusion, because both stand upon the same basis—consciousness. The *Yogi* says both are true; that we are bound so far as intelligence goes, that we are free as far as the soul is concerned. It is the real nature of man, the Soul, the *Purusa*, which is beyond all law of causation. Its freedom is percolating through layers and layers of matter, in various forms of intelligence, and mind, and all these things. It is its light which is shining through all. Intelligence has no light of its own. Each organ has a particular centre in the brain; it is not that all the organs have one centre; each organ is separate. Why do all these perceptions harmonise, and where do they get their unity? If it were in the brain there would be one centre only for the eyes, the nose, the ears, while we know for certain that there are different centres for each. But a man can see and hear at the same time, so a unity must be back of intelligence. Intelligence is eternally connected with the brain, but behind even intelligence stands the *Purusa*, the unit, where all these different sensations and perceptions join and become one. Soul itself is the centre where all the different organs converge and become unified, and that Soul is free, and it is its freedom that tells you every moment that you are free. But you mistake, and mingle that freedom every moment with intelligence and mind. You try to attribute that freedom to the intelligence, and immediately find that intelligence is not free; you attribute that freedom to the body, and immediately nature tells you that you are again mistaken. That is why there is this mingled sense of freedom and bondage at the same time. The *Yogi* analyses both what is free and what is bound, and his ignorance vanishes. He finds that the *Purusa* is free, is the essence of that knowledge which, coming through the *Buddhi*, becomes intelligence, and, as such, is bound.

21

तदर्थ एव दृश्यस्यात्मा

tad-artha eva dṛśyasyātmā

The nature of the experience is for him.

Nature has no light of its own. As long as the *Purusa* is present in it, it appears light, but the light is borrowed; just as the moon's light is reflected. All the manifestations of nature are caused by this nature itself, according to the *Yogis*; but nature has no purpose in view, except to free the *Purusa*.

22

कृतार्थं प्रति नष्टमप्यनष्टं तदन्यसाधारणत्वात्

kṛtārthaṃ prati naṣṭam-apyanaṣṭaṃ tad-anya-sādhāraṇatvāt

> Though destroyed for him whose goal has been gained, yet is not destroyed, being common to others.

The whole idea of this nature is to make the Soul know that it is entirely separate from nature, and when the Soul knows this, nature has no more attractions for it. But the whole of nature vanishes only for that man who has become free. There will always remain an infinite number of others, for whom nature will go on working.

23

स्वस्वामिशक्त्योः स्वरूपोपलब्धिहेतुः संयोगः

sva-svāmi-śaktyoḥ svarūpoplabdhi-hetuḥ saṃyogaḥ

> Junction is the cause of the realisation of the nature of both the powers, the experienced and its Lord.

According to this aphorism, when this Soul comes into conjunction with nature, both the power of the Soul and the power of nature become manifest in this conjunction, and all these manifestations are thrown out. Ignorance is the cause of this conjunction. We see every day that the cause of our pain or pleasure is always our joining ourselves with the body. If I were perfectly certain that I am not this body, I should take no notice of heat and cold, or anything of the kind. This body is a combination. It is only a fiction to say that I have one body, you another, and the sun another. The whole universe is one ocean of matter, and you are the name of a little particle, and I of another, and the sun of another. We know that this matter is continuously changing, what is forming the sun one day, the next day may form the matter of our bodies.

24

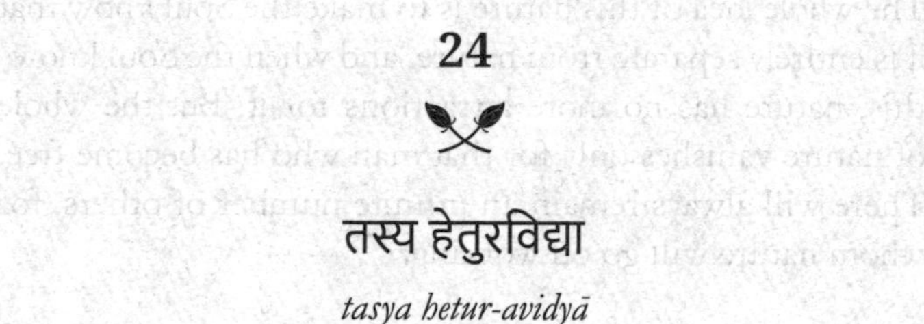

तस्य हेतुरविद्या

tasya hetur-avidyā

Ignorance is its cause.

Through ignorance we have joined ourselves with a particular body, and thus opened ourselves to misery. This idea of body is a simple superstition. It is superstition that makes us happy or unhappy. It is superstition caused by ignorance that makes us feel heat and cold, pain and pleasure. It is our business to rise above this superstition, and the *Yogi* shows us how we can do this. It has been demonstrated that, under certain mental conditions, a man may be burned, yet, while that condition lasts, he will feel no pain. The difficulty is that this sudden upheaval of the mind comes like a whirlwind one minute, and goes away the next. If, however, we attain it scientifically, through *Yoga*, we shall permanently attain to that separation of Self from the body.

25

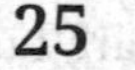

तदभावात् संयोगाभावो हानं तद्दृशेः कैवल्यम्

tad-abhābāt saṃyogābhāvo hānaṃ tad-dṛśeḥ kaivalyam

There being absence of that (ignorance) there is absence of junction, which is the thing-to-be-avoided; that is the independence of the seer.

According to this *Yoga* philosophy it is through ignorance that the Soul has been joined with nature and the idea is to get rid of nature's control over us. That is the goal of all religions. Each Soul is potentially divine. The goal is to manifest this Divinity within, by controlling nature, external and internal. Do this either by work, or worship, or psychic control, or by philosophy, by one, or more, or all of these—and be free. This is the whole of religion. Doctrines, or dogmas, or rituals, or books, or temples, or forms, are but secondary details. The *Yogi* tries to reach this goal through psychic control. Until we can free ourselves from nature we are slaves; as she dictates so we must go. The *Yogi* claims that he who controls mind controls matter also.

The internal nature is much higher that the external, and much more difficult to grapple with, much more difficult to control; therefore he who has conquered the internal nature controls the whole universe; it becomes his servant. *Rāja Yoga* propounds the methods of gaining this control. Higher forces than we know in physical nature will have to be subdued. This body is just the external crust of the mind. They are not two different things; they are just as the oyster and its shell. They are but two aspects of one thing; the internal substance of the oyster is taking up matter from outside, and manufacturing the shell. In the same way these internal fine forces which are called mind take up gross matter from outside, and from that manufacture this external shell, or body. If then, we have control of the internal, it is very easy to have control of the external. Then again, these forces are not different. It is not that some forces are physical, and some mental; the physical forces are but the gross manifestations of the fine forces, just as the physical world is but the gross manifestation of the fine world.

26

विवेकख्यातिरविप्लवा हानोपायः

viveka-khyātir-aviplavā hānopāyaḥ

> The means of destruction of ignorance is unbroken practice of discrimination.

This is the real goal of practice—discrimination between the real and unreal, knowing that the *Purusa* is not nature, that it is neither matter nor mind, and that because it is not nature, it cannot possibly change. It is only nature which changes, combining, and recombining, dissolving continually. When through constant practice we begin to discriminate, ignorance will vanish, and the *Purusa* will begin to shine in its real nature, omniscient, omnipotent, omnipresent.

27

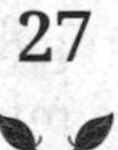

तस्य सप्तधा प्रान्तभूमिः प्रज्ञा

tasya saptadhā prānta-bhūmiḥ prajñā

His knowledge is of the sevenfold highest ground.

When this knowledge comes, it will come, as it were, in seven grades, one after the other, and when one of these has begun we may know that we are getting knowledge. The first to appear will be that we have known what is to be known. The mind will cease to be dissatisfied. While we are aware of thirsting after knowledge we begin to seek here and there, wherever we think we can get some truth, and, failing to find it we become dissatisfied and seek in a fresh direction. All search is vain, until we begin to perceive that knowledge is within ourselves, that no one can help us, that we must help ourselves. When we begin to practice the power of discrimination, the first sign that we are getting near truth will be that that dissatisfied state will vanish. We shall feel quite sure that we have found the truth, and that it cannot be anything else but the truth. Then we may know that the sun is rising, that the morning is breaking for us, and, taking courage, we must persevere until the goal is reached. The second grade will be that all pains will be gone. It will be impossible for anything in the universe, physical, mental, or spiritual, to give us pain. The third will be that we shall get full knowledge, that omniscience will be ours. Next will come what is called freedom of the *Chitta*. We shall realise that all these difficulties and struggles have fallen off from us. All these vacillations of the mind, when the mind cannot be controlled, have fallen down, just as a stone falls from the mountain top into the valley and never comes up again. The next will be that this *Chitta* itself will realise that it melts away into its causes whenever we so desire. Lastly we shall find that we are established in our Self, that we have been alone throughout the universe, neither body nor mind was ever connected with us, much less joined to us. They were working their own way, and we, through ignorance, joined ourselves to them. But we have been alone, omnipotent, omnipresent, ever blessed; our own Self was so pure and perfect that we required none else. We required none else to make us happy, for we are happiness itself. We shall find that this knowledge does not depend on anything else; throughout the universe there can be nothing that will not become effulgent before our knowledge. This will be the last state, and the *Yogi* will become peaceful and calm, never to feel any more pain, never to be again deluded, never to touch misery. He knows he is ever blessed, ever perfect, almighty.

28

योगाङ्गानुष्ठानादशुद्धिक्षये ज्ञानदीप्तिराविवेकख्यातेः

yogāṅgānuṣṭhānād-aśuddhi-kṣaye jñāna-dīptir-āviveka-khyāteḥ

By the practice of the different parts of Yoga the impurities being destroyed knowledge becomes effulgent, up to discrimination.

Now comes the practical knowledge. What we have just been speaking about is much higher. It is way above our heads, but it is the ideal. It is first necessary to obtain physical and mental control. Then the realisation will become steady in that ideal. The ideal being known, what remains is to practise the method of reaching it.

29

यमनियमासनप्राणायामप्रत्याहारधारणाध्यान-समाधयोऽष्टाव अङ्गानि

yama-niyamāsana-prāṇāyāma-pratyāhāra-dhāraṇā-dhyāna-samādhayo'ṣṭāv-aṅgāni

Yama, *Niyama*, *Āsana*, *Prānāyāma*, *Pratyāhāra*, *Dhāranā*, *Dhyāna*, *Samādhi*, are the limbs of *Yoga*.

30

अहिंसासत्यास्तेयब्रह्मचर्यापरिग्रहा यमाः

ahiṃsā-satyāsteya-brahmacaryāparigrahā yamāḥ

Non-killing, truthfulness, non-stealing, continence, and non-receiving, are called *Yama.*

A man who wants to be a perfect *Yogi* must give up the sex idea. The Soul has no sex; why should it degrade itself with sex ideas? Later we shall understand better why these ideas must be given up. Receiving is just as bad as stealing; receiving gifts from others. Whoever receives gifts, his mind is acted on by the mind of the giver, so that the man who receives gifts becomes degenerated. Receiving gifts destroys the independence of the mind, and makes us mere slaves. Therefore, receive nothing.

31

जातिदेशकालसमयानवच्छिन्नाः
सार्वभौमा महाव्रतम्

jāti-deśa-kāla-samayānavacchinnāḥ
sārvabhaumā-mahāvratam

These, unbroken by time, place, purpose, and caste, are (universal) great vows.

These practices, non-killing, non-stealing, chastity, and non-receiving, are to be practiced by every man, woman and child, by every soul, irrespective of nation, country or position.

32

शौचसंतोषतपःस्वाध्यायेश्वरप्रणिधानानि नियमाः

śauca-santoṣa-tapaḥ-svādhyāyeśvara-praṇidhānāni niyamāḥ

> Internal and external purification, contentment, mortification, study, and worship of God, are the *Niyamas.*

External purification is keeping the body pure; a dirty man will never become a *Yogi*. There must be internal purification also. That is obtained by the first-named virtues. Of course internal purity is of greater value that external, but both are necessary, and external purity, without internal, is of no good.

33

वितर्कबाधने प्रतिपक्षभावनम्

vitarka-bādhane pratiprakṣa-bhāvanam

> To obstruct thoughts which are inimical to *Yoga* contrary thoughts will be brought.

This is the way to practice all these virtues that have been stated, by holding thoughts of an opposite character in the mind. When the idea of stealing comes, non-stealing should be thought of. When the idea of receiving gifts comes, replace it by a contrary thought.

34

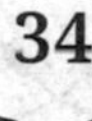

वितर्का हिंसादयः कृतकारितानुमोदिता लोभक्रोधमोहपूर्वका मृदुमध्याधिमात्रा दुःखाज्ञानानन्तफला इति प्रतिपक्षभावनम्

vitarkā hiṃsādayaḥ kṛta-kāritānumoditā lobha-krodha-mohāpūrvakā mṛdu-madhyādhimātrā duḥkhājñānānanta-phalā iti pratiprakṣa-bhāvanam

> The obstructions to *Yoga* are killing etc., whether committed, caused, or approved; either through avarice, or anger, or ignorance; whether slight, middling, or great, and result is innumerable ignorance and miseries. This is (the method of) thinking the contrary.

If I tell I lie, or cause another to tell a lie, or approve of another doing so, it is equally sinful. If it is a very mild lie, it is still a lie. Every vicious thought will rebound, every thought of hatred which you have thought, in a cave even, is stored up, and will one day come back to you with tremendous power in the form of some misery here. If you project all sorts of hatred and jealousy, they will rebound on you with compound interest. No power can avert them; when once you have put them in motion you will have to bear them. Remembering this, will prevent you from doing wicked things.

35

अहिंसाप्रतिष्ठायां तत्सन्निधौ वैरत्यागः

ahiṃsā-pratiṣṭhāyaṃ tat-sannidhau vairatyāghaḥ

Non-killing being established, in his presence all enmities cease (in others).

If a man gets the idea of non-injuring others, before him even animals which are by their nature ferocious will become peaceful. The tiger and the lamb will play together before that *Yogi* and will not hurt each other. When you have come to that state, then alone you will understand that you have become firmly established in non-injuring.

36

सत्यप्रतिष्ठायां क्रियाफलाश्रयत्वम्

satya-pratiṣṭthāyaṃ kriyā-phalāśrayatvam

By the establishment of truthfulness the *Yogi* gets the power of attaining for himself and others the fruits of work without the works.

When this power of truth will be established with you, then even in dream you will never tell an untruth, in thought, word or deed; whatever you say will be truth. You may say to a man "Be blessed," and that man will be blessed. If a man is diseased, and you say to him, "Be thou cured," he will be cured immediately.

37

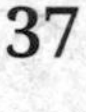

अस्तेयप्रतिष्ठायां सर्वरत्नोपस्थानम्

asteya-pratiṣṭhāyāṃ sarva-ratnopasthānam

> By the establishment of non-stealing all wealth comes to the *Yogi*.

The more you fly from nature the more she follows you, and if you do not care for her at all she becomes your slave.

38

ब्रह्मचर्यप्रतिष्ठायां वीर्यलाभः

brahma-carya pratiṣṭhāyāṃ vīrya-lābhaḥ

> By the establishment of continence energy is gained.

The chaste brain has tremendous energy, gigantic will power, without that there can be no mental strength. All men of gigantic brains are very continent. It gives wonderful control over mankind. Leaders of men have been very continent, and this is what gave them power. Therefore the *Yogi* must be continent.

39

अपरिग्रहस्थैर्ये जन्मकथन्तसंबोधः

aparigraha-sthairye janma-kathantā-saṃbodhaḥ

> When he is fixed in non-receiving he gets the memory of past life.

When the *Yogi* does not receive presents from others he does not become beholden to others, but becomes independent and free, and his mind becomes pure, because with every gift he receives all the evils of the giver, and they come and lay coating after coating on his mind, until it is hidden under all sorts of coverings of evil. If he does not receive the mind becomes pure, and the first thing it gets is memory of past life.

Then alone the *Yogi* becomes perfectly fixed in his ideal, because he sees that he has been coming and going so many times, and he becomes determined that this time he will be free, that he will no more come and go, and be the slave of Nature.

40

शौचात्स्वङ्गजुगुप्सा परैरसंसर्गः

śaucāt svāṅga-jugupsā parair-asaṃsargaḥ

Internal and external cleanliness being established, arises disgust for one's own body, and non-intercourse with other bodies.

When there is real purification of the body, external and internal, there arises neglect of the body, and all this idea of keeping it nice will vanish. What others call the most beautiful face to the *Yogi* will appear to be an animal's face, if there is not intelligence behind it. What the world will call a very common face he will call heavenly, if that spirit shines behind it. This thirst after body is the great bane of human life. So, when this purity is established, the first sign will be that you do not care to think you are a body. It is only when purity comes that we get rid of this body idea.

41

सत्त्वशुद्धिसौमनस्यैकाग्र्येन्द्रियजयात्मदर्शनयोग्यत्वानि च

sattva-śuddhiḥ-saumanasyaikāgryendriya-jayātma-darśana-yogyatvāni ca

There also arises purification of the *Sattva*, cheerfulness of the mind, concentration, conquest of the organs, and fitness for the realisation of the Self.

By this practice the *Sattva* material will prevail, and the mind will become concentrated and cheerful. The first sign that you are become religious is that you are becoming cheerful. When a man is gloomy that may be dyspepsia, but it is not religion. A pleasurable feeling is the nature of the *Sattva*. Everything is pleasurable to the *Sāttvika* man, and when this comes, know that you are progressing in *Yoga*. All pain is caused by *Tamas*, so you must get rid of that; moroseness is one of the results of *Tamas*. The strong, the well-knit, the young, the healthy, the daring alone are fit to be *Yogis*. To the *Yogi* everything is bliss, every human face that he sees brings cheerfulness to him. That is the sign of a virtuous man. Misery is caused by sin, and by no other cause. What business have you with clouded faces; it is terrible. If you have a clouded face do not go out that day, shut yourself up in your room. What right have you to carry this disease out into the world? When your mind has become controlled you will have control over the whole body; instead of being a slave to the machine, the machine will be your slave. Instead of this machine being able to drag the soul down it will be its greatest helpmate.

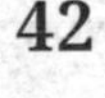

सन्तोषादनुत्तमः सुखलाभः

santoṣāt-anuttamaḥ sukha-lābhaḥ

From contentment comes superlative happiness.

43

कायेन्द्रियसिद्धिरशुद्धिक्षयात् तपसः

kāyendriya-siddhir-aśuddhi-kṣayāt tapasaḥ

The result of mortification is bringing powers to the organs and the body, by destroying the impurity.

The results of mortification are seen immediately sometimes by heightened powers of vision, and so on, hearing things at a distance, etc.

44

स्वाध्यायादिष्टदेवतासम्प्रयोगः

svādhyāyād-iṣṭa-devatā samprayogaḥ

By repetition of the *mantra* comes the realisation of the intended deity.

The higher the beings that you want to get the harder is the practice.

45

समाधिसिद्धिरीश्वरप्रणिधानात्

samādhi-siddhir-Īśvara-praṇidhānāt

By sacrificing all to *Isvara* comes *Samādhi.*

By resignation to the Lord, *Samādhi* becomes perfect.

46

स्थिरसुखमासनम्

sthira-sukham-āsanam

Posture is that which is firm and pleasant.

Now comes *Āsana*, posture. Until you can get a firm seat you cannot practice the breathing and other exercises. The seat being firm means that you do not feel the body at all; then alone it has become firm. But, in the ordinary way, you will find that as soon as you sit for a few minutes all sorts of disturbances come into the body; but when you have got beyond the idea of a concrete body you will lose all sense of the body. You will feel neither pleasure nor pain. And when you take your body up again it will feel so rested; it is the only perfect rest that you can give to the body. When you have succeeded in conquering the body and keeping it firm, your practice will remain firm, but while you are disturbed by the body your nerves become disturbed, and you cannot concentrate the mind. We can make the seat firm by thinking of the infinite. We cannot think of the Absolute Infinite, but we can think of the infinite sky

47

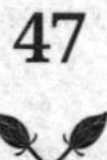

प्रयत्नशैथिल्यानन्तसमापत्तिभ्याम्

prayatna-śaithilyānanta-samāpattibhyām

By slight effort and meditating on the unlimited (posture becomes firm and pleasant).

Light and darkness, pleasure and pain, will not then disturb you.

48

ततो द्वन्द्वानभिघातः

tato dvandvānabhighātaḥ

Seat being conquered, the dualities do not obstruct.

The dualities are good and bad, heat and cold, and all the pairs of opposites.

49

तस्मिन् सति श्वासप्रश्वासयोर्गतिविच्छेदः प्राणायामः

tasmin sati śvāsa-praśvāsyor gati-vicchedaḥ prāṇāyāmaḥ

> Controlling the motion of the exhalation and the inhalation follows after this.

When the posture has been conquered, then this motion is to be broken and controlled, and thus we come to Prānāyāma; the controlling of the vital forces of the body. *Prāna* is not breath, though it is usually so translated. It is the sum-total of the cosmic energy. It is the energy that is in each body, and its most apparent manifestation is the motion of the lungs. This motion is caused by *Prāna* drawing in the breath, and is what we seek to control in *Prānāyāma*. We begin by controlling the breath, as the easiest way of getting control of the *Prāna*.

50

बाह्याभ्यन्तरस्तम्भवृत्तिर्देशकालसंख्याभिः
परिदृष्टो दीर्घसूक्ष्मः

bāhyābhyantara-sthambha-vṛttir-deśa-kāla-sankhyābhiḥ
paridṛṣṭo dīrgha-sūkṣmaḥ

> Its modifications are either external or internal, or motionless, regulated by place, time, and number, either long or short.

The three sorts of motion of this *Prānāyāma* are, one by which we draw the breath in, another by which we throw it out, and the third action is when the breath is held in the lungs, or stopped from entering the lungs. These, again, are varied by place and time. By place is meant that the *Prāna* is held to some particular part of the body. By time is meant how long the *Prāna* should be confined to a certain place, and so we are told how many seconds to keep on motion, and how many seconds to keep another. The result of this *Prānāyāma* is *Udghāta*, awakening the *Kundalini*.

51

बाह्याभ्यन्तरविषयाक्षेपी चतुर्थः

bāhyābhyantara-viṣayākṣepī caturthaḥ

> The fourth is restraining the *Prāna* by directing it either to the external or internal objects.

This is the fourth sort of *Prānāyāma*. *Prāna* can be directed either inside or outside.

52

ततः क्षीयते प्रकाशावरणम्

tataḥ kṣīyate prakāśāvaraṇam

> From that, the covering to the light of the *Chitta* is attenuated.

The *Chitta* has, by its own nature, all knowledge. It is made of *Sattva* particles, but is covered by *Rajas* and *Tamas* particles, and by *Prānāyāma* this covering is removed.

53

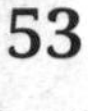

धारणासु च योग्यता मनसः

dhāraṇāsu ca yogyatā manasaḥ

> The mind becomes fit for *Dhāraṇā*.

After this covering has been removed we are able to concentrate the mind.

54

स्वविषयासम्प्रयोगे चित्तस्य स्वरूपानुकार इवेन्द्रियाणां प्रत्याहारः

sva-viṣayāsamprayoge cittasya svarūpānukāra ivendriyāṇāṃ pratyāhāraḥ

> The drawing in of the organs is by their giving up their own objects and taking the form of the mind-stuff.

These organs are separate states of the mind-stuff. I see a book; the form is not in the book, it is in the mind. Something is outside which calls that form up. The real form is in the *Chitta*. These organs are identifying themselves with, and taking the forms of whatever comes to them. If you can restrain the mind-stuff from taking these forms the mind will remain calm. This is called *Pratyāhāra*.

55

ततः परमा वश्यतेन्द्रियाणाम्

tataḥ paramā-vaśyatā indriyāṇām

Thence arises supreme control of the organs.

When the *Yogi* has succeeded in preventing the organs from taking the forms of external objects, and in making them remain one with the mind-stuff, then comes perfect control of the organs, and when the organs are perfectly under control, every muscle and nerve will be under control, because the organs are the centres of all the sensations, and of all actions. These organs are divided into organs of work and organs of sensation. When the organs are controlled the *Yogi* can control all feeling and doing; the whole of the body will be under his control. Then alone one begins to feel joy in being born; then one can truthfully say, "Blessed am I that I was born." When that control of the organs is obtained, we feel how wonderful this body really is.

PART III

VIBHŪTI PADA

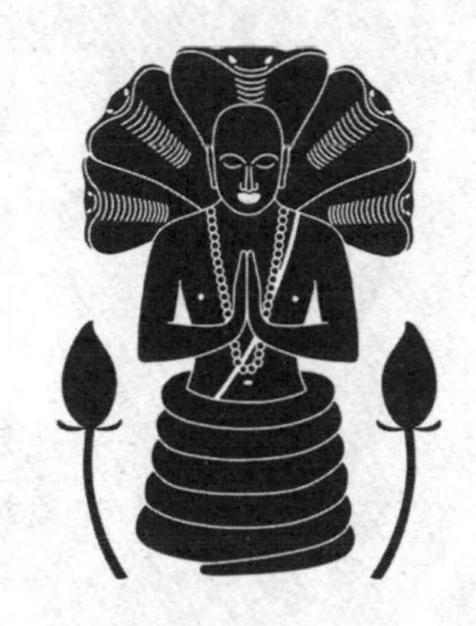

The Chapter of Powers

॥ तृतीयः विभूतिपादः ॥

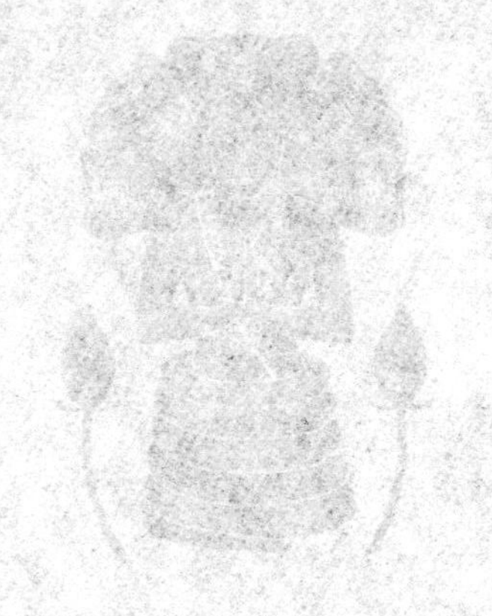

1

देशबन्धश्चित्तस्य धारणा

deśa-bandhaś cittasya dhāraṇā

> *Dhāranā* is holding the mind on to some particular object.

Dhāranā (concentration) is when the mind holds on to some object, either in the body, or outside the body, and keeps itself in that state.

2

तत्र प्रत्ययैकतानता ध्यानम्

tatra pratyaya-ikatānatā dhyānam

> An unbroken flow of knowledge to that object is *Dhyāna*.

The mind tries to think of one object, to hold itself to one particular spot, as the top of the head, the heart, etc., and if the mind succeeds in receiving the sensations only through that part of the body, and through no other part, that would be *Dhāranā*, and when the mind succeeds in keeping itself in that state for some time it is called *Dhyāna* (meditation).

3

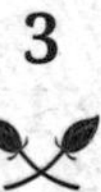

तदेवार्थ मात्रनिर्भासं स्वरूपशून्यमिवसमाधिः

tad-evārtha mātra-nirbhāsaṃ svarūpa-śūnyam-iva-samādhiḥ

> When that, giving up all forms, reflects only the meaning, it is *Samādhi.*

That is, when in meditation all forms are given up. Suppose I were meditating on a book, and that I have gradually succeeded in concentrating the mind on it, and perceiving only the internal sensations, the meaning, unexpressed in any form, that state of *Dhyāna* is called *Samādhi.*

4

त्रयमेकत्र संयमः

trayam-ekatra saṃyamaḥ

> (These) three (when practised) in regard to one object is *Samyama.*

When a man can direct his mind to any particular object

and fix it there, and then keep it there for a long time, separating the object from the internal part, this is *Samyama*; or *Dhāranā*, *Dhyāna*, and *Samādhi*, one following the other, and making one. The form of the thing has vanished, and only its meaning remains in the mind.

5

तज्जयात् प्रज्ञालोकः

tajjayāt prajñālokaḥ

By the conquest of that comes light of knowledge.

When one has succeeded in making this *Samyama*, all powers come under his control. This is the great instrument of the *Yogi*. The object of knowledge are infinite, and they are divided into the gross, grosser, grossest, and the fine, finer, finest, and so on. This *Samyama* should be first applied to gross things, when you begin to get knowledge of the gross, slowly, by stages, it should be brought to finer things.

6

तस्य भूमिषु विनियोगः

tasya bhūmiṣu viniyogaḥ

That should be employed in stages.

This is a note of warning not to attempt to go too fast.

7

त्रयमन्तरङ्गम् पूर्वेभ्यः

trayam-antar-angam pūrvebhyaḥ

These three are nearer than those that precede.

Before these we had the *Prānāyāma*, the *Āsana*, the *Yama* and *Niyama*; these are external parts of these three—*Dhāranā*, *Dhyāna*, and *Samādhi*. Yet these latter even are external to the seedless *Samādhi*. When a man has attained to them he may attain to omniscience and omnipresence, but that would not be salvation. These three would not make the mind *Nirvikalpa*, changeless, but would leave the seeds for getting bodies again; only when the seeds are, as the *Yogi* says, "fried," do they lose the possibility of producing further plants. These powers cannot fry the seed.

8

तदपि बहिरङ्गंम्निर्बीजस्य

tadapi bahiraṅgam nirbījasya

But even they are external to the seedless (*Samādhi*).

Compared with that seedless *Samādhi*, therefore, even these are external. We have not yet reached the real *Samādhi*, the highest, but to a lower stage, in which this universe still exists as we see it, and in which are all these power.

9

व्युत्थाननिरोधसंस्कारयोरभिभवप्रादुर्भावौ निरोधक्षणचित्तान्वयो निरोधपरिणामः

vyutthāna-nirodha-saṃskārayor-abhibhava prādurbhāvau nirodha-kṣaṇa-cittānvayo nirodha-pariṇāmaḥ

> By the suppression of the disturbed modifications of the mind, and by the rise of modifications of control, the mind is said to attain the controlling modifications—following the controlling powers of the mind.

That is to say, in this first state of *Samādhi*, the modifications of the mind have been controlled, but not perfectly, because if they were, there would be no modifications. If there is a modification which impels the mind to rush out through the senses, and the *Yogi* tries to control it, that very control itself will be a modification. One wave will be checked by another wave, so it will not be real *Samādhi*, when all the waves have subsided, as control itself will be a wave. Yet this lower *Samādhi* is very much nearer to the higher *Samādhi* than when the mind comes bubbling out.

10

तस्य प्रशान्तवाहिता संस्कारात्

tasya praśānta-vāhitā saṃskārat

Its flow becomes steady by habit.

The flow of this continuous control of the mind becomes steady when practices day after day and the mind obtains the faculty of constant concentration.

11

सर्वार्थतैकाग्रतयोः क्षयोदयौ चित्तस्य समाधिपरिणमः

sarvārthatā ekāgrātayoḥ kṣayodayau cittasya samādhi-pariṇāmaḥ

> Taking in all sorts of objects and concentrating upon one object, these two powers being destroyed and manifested respectively, the *Chitta* gets the modification called *Samādhi*.

The mind is taking up various objects, running into all sorts of things and then there is a higher state of the mind, when it takes up one object and excludes all others. *Samādhi* is the result of that.

12

ततः पुनःशान्तोदितौ तुल्यप्रत्ययौ
चित्तस्यैकाग्रतापरिणामः

tataḥ punaḥśātoditau tulya-pratyayau
cittasyaikāgratā-pariṇāmaḥ

The one-pointedness of the *Chitta* is when it grasps in one, the past and present.

How are we to know that the mind has become concentrated? Because time will vanish. The more time vanishes the more concentrated we are. In common life we see that when were are interested in a book we do not note the time at all, and when we leave the book we are often surprised to find how many hours have passed. All time will have the tendency to come and stand in the one present. So the definition is given, when the past and present come and stand in one, the more concentrated the mind.

13

एतेन भूतेन्द्रियेषु धर्मलक्षणावस्थापरिणामा व्याख्याताः

etena bhūtendriyeṣu dharma-lakṣaṇāvasthā-pariṇāmā vyākhyātāḥ

By this is explained the threefold transformations of form, time, and state, in fine or gross matter, and in the organs.

By this the threefold changes in the mind-stuff as to form, time, and state are explained. The mind-stuff is changing into *Vrttis*, this is change as to form. To be able to hold the changes to the present time is change as to time. To be able to make the mind-stuff go to the past forms giving up the present even, is change as to state. The concentrations taught in the preceding aphorisms were to give the *Yogi* a voluntary control over the transformations of his mind-stuff which alone will enable him to make the *Samyama* before named.

14

शान्तोदिताव्यपदेश्यधर्मानुपाति धर्मि

śānoditāvyapadeśya-dharmānupātī dharmī

That which is acted upon by transformations,

either past, present or yet to be manifested, is the qualified.

That is to say, the qualified is the substance which is being acted upon by time and by the *Samskāras*, and getting changed and being manifested all the time.

15

क्रमान्यत्वाम् परिणामान्यत्वे हेतुः

kramānyatvaṃ pariṇāmānyateve hetuḥ

The succession of changes is the cause of manifold evolution.

16

परिणाम त्रय संयमादतीतानागतज्ञानम्

pariṇāma traya saṃyamāt-atītānāgata-jñānam

By making *Samyama* on the three sorts of changes comes the knowledge of past and future.

We must not lose sight of the first definition of *Samyama*. When the mind has attained to that state when it identifies itself with the internal impression of the object, leaving the external, and when, by long practice, that is retained by the mind, and the mind can get into that state in a moment, that is *Samyama*. If a man in that state wants to know the past and future he has to make a *Samyama* on the changes in the *Samskāras*. Some are working now at present, some have worked out, and some are waiting to work; so by making a *Samyama* on these he knows the past and future.

17

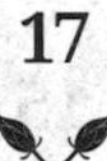

शब्दार्थप्रत्ययानामितरेतराध्यासात्सङ्करस्तत्प्रविभागसंयमात्
सर्वभूतरुतज्ञानम्

śabdārtha-pratyayāmām-itaretarādhyāsāt-saṅkaras-tat-pravibhāga-saṃyamāt sarva-bhūta-ruta-jñānam

> By making *Samyama* on word, meaning, and knowledge, which are ordinarily confused, comes the knowledge of all animal sounds.

The word represents the external cause, the meaning represents the internal vibration that travels to the brain through the channels of the *Indriyas*, conveying the external impression to the mind, and knowledge represents the reaction of the mind, with which comes perception. These three confused, make our sense objects. Suppose I hear a word; there is first the external vibration, next the internal sensation carried to the mind by the organ of hearing, then the mind reacts, and I know the word. The word I know is a mixture of the three, vibration, sensation, and reaction. Ordinarily these three are inseparable; but by practice the *Yogi* can separate them.

When a man has attained to this, if he makes a *Samyama* on any sound, he understands the meaning which that sound was intended to express, whether it was made by man or by any other animal.

18

संस्कारसाक्षात्करणात् पूर्वजातिज्ञानम्

saṃskāra-sākṣāt-karaṇāt pūrva-jāti-jñānam

By perceiving the impressions, knowledge of past life.

Each experience that we have comes in the form of a wave in the *Chitta*, and this subsides and becomes finer and finer, but is never lost. It remains there in minute form, and if we can bring this wave up again, it becomes memory. So, if the *Yogi* can make a *Samyama* on these past impressions in the mind, he will begin to remember all his past lives.

19

प्रत्ययस्य परचित्तज्ञानम्

pratyayasya para-citta-jñānam

By making *Samyama* on the signs in another's both knowledge of that mind comes.

Suppose each man has particular signs on his body, which differentiate him from others; when the *Yogi* makes a *Samyama* on these signs peculiar to a certain man he knows the nature of the mind of that person.

20

न च तत् सालम्बनं तस्याविषयीभूतत्वात्

na ca tat sālambanaṃ tasyāviṣayī-bhūtatvāt

> But not its contents, that not being the object of the *Samyama*.

He would not know the contents of the mind by making a *Samyama* on the body. There would be required a twofold *Samyama*, first on the signs in the body, and then on the mind itself. The *Yogi* would then know everything that is in that mind, past, present, and future.

21

कायरूपसंयमात् तद्ग्राह्याशक्तिस्तम्भे
चक्षुःप्रकाशासम्प्रयोगेऽन्तर्धानम्

kāya-rūpa-saṃyamāt tat-grāhya-śakti-stambhe
cakṣuḥ prakāśāsamprayoge'ntardhānam

> By making *Samyama* on the form of the body the power of perceiving forms being obstructed, the power of manifestation in the eye being separated, the *Yogi*'s body becomes unseen.

A *Yogi* standing in the midst of this room can apparently vanish. He does not really vanish, but he will not be seen by anyone. The form and the body are, as it were, separated. You must remember that this can only be done when the *Yogi* has attained to that power of concentration when form and the thing formed have been separated. Then he makes a *Samyama* on that, and the power to perceive forms is obstructed, because the power of perceiving forms comes from the junction of form and the thing formed.

22

एतेन शब्दाद्यन्तर्धानमुक्तम्

etena śhabdādyantardhānam uktam

> By this the disappearance or concealment of words which are being spoken is also explained.

23

सोपक्रमं निरुपक्रमं च कर्म
तत्संयमादपरान्तज्ञानमरिष्टेभ्यो वा

sopakramaṃ nirupakramaṃ ca karma tat-saṃyamād-aparānta-jñānam-ariṣṭebhyo vā

> *Karma* is of two kinds, soon to be fructified, and late to be fructified. By making *Samyama* on that, or by the signs called *Aristha*, portents, the Yogis know the exact time of separation from their bodies.

When the *Yogi* makes a *Samyama* on his own *Karma*, upon those impressions in his mind which are now working, and those which are just waiting to work, he knows exactly by those that are waiting when his body will fall. He knows when he will die, at what hour, even at what minute. The Hindus think very much of that knowledge or consciousness of the nearness of death, because it is taught in the Gitā that the thoughts at the moment of departure are great powers in determining the next life.

24

मैत्र्यादिषु बलानि

maitryādiṣu balāni

By making *Samyama* on friendship, etc., various strength comes.

25

बलेषु हस्तिबलादीनि

baleṣu hasti-balādīnī

By making *Samyama* on the strength of the elephant, etc., that strength comes to the *Yogi.*

When a *Yogi* has attained to this *Samyama* and wants strength, he makes a *Samyama* on the strength of the elephant, and gets it. Infinite energy is at the disposal of everyone, if he only knows how to get it. The *Yogi* has discovered the science of getting it.

26

प्रवृत्त्यालोकन्यासात् सूक्ष्मव्यवहितविप्रकृष्टज्ञानम्

pravṛttyāloka-nyāsāt sūkṣmā-vyāvahita-viprakṛṣṭa-jñānam

By making *Samyama* on that effulgent light comes the knowledge of the fine, the obstructed, and the remote.

When the *Yogi* makes *Samyama* on that effulgent light in the heart he sees things which are very remote, things, for instance, that are happening in a distant place, and which are obstructed by mountain barriers and also things which are very fine.

27

भुवनज्ञानं सूर्ये संयमात्

bhuvana-jñānaṃ sūrye saṃyamāt

By making *Samyama* on the sun, (comes) the knowledge of the world.

28

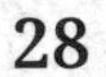

चन्द्रे ताराव्यूहज्ञानम्

candre tāra-vyūha-jñānam

On the moon, (comes) the knowledge of the cluster of stars.

29

ध्रुवे तद्गतिज्ञानम्

dhruve tad-gati-jñānam

On the pole star (comes) the knowledge of the motions of the stars.

30

नाभिचक्रे कायव्यूहज्ञानम्

nābhi-cakre kāya-vyūha-jñānam

On the navel circle (comes) the knowledge of the constitution of the body.

31

कण्ठकूपे क्षुत्पिपासानिवृत्तिः

kaṇṭha-kūpe kṣut-pipāsā-nivṛttiḥ

On the hollow of the throat (comes) cessation of hunger.

When a man is very hungry, if he can make *Samyama* on the pit of the throat hunger ceases.

32

कूर्मनाड्यां स्थैर्यम्

kūrma-nāḍyāṃ sthairyam

On the nerve called Kurma (comes) fixity of the body.

When he is practising the body is not disturbed.

33

मूर्धज्योतिषि सिद्धदर्शनम्

mūrdha-jyotiṣi siddha-darśanam

On the light emanating from the top of the head sight of the *Siddhas.*

The *Siddhas* are beings who are a little above ghosts. When the *Yogi* concentrates his mind on the top of his head he will see these *Siddhas.* The word *Siddha* does not refer to those men who have become free—a sense in which it is often used.

34

प्रतिभाद्वा सर्वम्

prātibhād-vā sarvam

Or by the power of *Pratibhā* all knowledge.

All these can come without any *Samyama* to the man who has the power of *Pratibhā* (enlightenment from purity). This is when a man has risen to a high state of *Pratibhā*; then he has that great light. All things are apparent to him. Everything comes to him naturally, without making *Samyama* on anything.

35

हृदये चित्तसंवित्

hṛaye citta-saṃvit

In the heart, knowledge of minds.

36

सत्त्वपुरुषयोरत्यन्तासङ्कीर्णयोः प्रत्ययाविशेषो
भोगः परार्थत्वात् स्वार्थसंयमात् पुरुषज्ञानम्

sattva-puruṣāyoratyantāsaṅkīrṇayoḥ pratyayāviśeṣo bhogaḥ parārthatvāt svārthasaṃyamāt puruṣajñānam

Enjoyment comes by the non-discrimination of the very distant soul and *Sattva.* Its actions are for another; *Samyama* on this gives knowledge of the *Purusa.*

All action of Sattva, a modification of Prakriti characterised by light and happiness, is for the soul. When Sattva is free from egoism and illuminated with the pure intelligence of Purusa, it is called the self-centred one, because in that state it becomes independent of all relations.

37

ततः प्रातिभश्रावणवेदनादर्शास्वादवार्ता जायन्ते

tataḥ prātibha-śrāvāṇa-vedanādarśāsvāda-vārtā jāyante

From that arises the knowledge of hearing, touching, seeing, tasting, and smelling, belonging to *Pratibhā*.

38

ते समाधावुपसर्गा व्युत्थाने सिद्धयः

te samādhāv upasargā vyutthāne siddhayaḥ

These are obstacles to *Samādhi*; but they are powers in the worldly state.

If the *Yogi* knows all these enjoyments of the world it comes by the junction of the *Purusa* and the mind. If he wants to make *Samyama* on this, that they are two different things, nature and soul, he gets knowledge of the *Purusa*. From that arises discrimination. When he has got that discrimination he gets the *Pratibhā*, the light of supreme genius. These powers, however, are obstructions to the attainment of the highest goal, the knowledge of the pure Self, and freedom; these are, as it were, to be met in the way, and if the *Yogi* rejects them, he attains the highest. If he is tempted to acquire these, his farther progress is barred.

39

बन्धकारणशैथिल्यात् प्रचारसंवेदनाच्च
चित्तस्य परशरीरावेशः

badnha-kāraṇa-śaithilyāt pracāra-saṃvedanāc ca
cittasya para-śarīrāveśaḥ

> When the cause of bondage has become loosened, the *Yogi*, by his knowledge of manifestation through the organs, enters another's body.

The *Yogi* can enter a dead body, and make it get up and move, even while he himself is working in another body. Or he can enter a living body, and hold that man's mind and organs in check, and for the time being act through the body of that man. That is done by the *Yogi* coming to this discrimination of *Purusa* and nature. If he wants to enter another's body he makes a *Samyama* on that body and enters it, because, not only is his Soul omnipresent, but his mind also, according to the *Yogi*. It is one bit of the universal mind. Now, however, it can only work through the nerve currents in this body, but when the *Yogi* has loosened himself from these nerve currents, he will be able to work through other things.

40

उदानजयाज्जलपङ्कण्टकादिष्वसङ्ग उत्क्रान्तिश् च

udāna-jayāj jala-paṅkha-kaṇṭakādiṣvasaṅgo utkrāntiś ca

By conquering the current called *Udana* the *Yogi* does not sink in water, or in swamps, and he can walk on thorns etc., and can die at will.

Udana is the name of the nerve current that governs the lungs, and all the upper parts of the body, and when he is master of it he becomes light in weight. He cannot sink in water; he can walk on thorns and sword blades, and stand in fire, and so on.

41

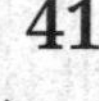

समानजयाज्ज्वलनम्

samāna-jayāj-jvalanam

By the conquest of the current *Samana* he is surrounded by blaze.

Whenever he likes light flashes from his body.

42

श्रोत्राकाशयोः सम्बन्धसंयमाद्दिव्यं श्रोत्रम्

śrotrākāśayoḥ sambandha-saṃyamād-divyaṃ śrotram

By making *Samyama* on the relation between the ear and the *Ākāsa* comes divine hearing.

There is the *Ākāsa*, the ether, and the instrument, the ear. By making *Samyama* on them the *Yogi* gets divine hearing; he hears everything. Anything spoken or sounded miles away he can here.

43

कायाकाशयोः सम्बन्धसंयमाल्लघुतूलसमापत्तेश्
चाकाशगमनम्

kāyākāśayoḥ sambandha-saṃyamāl-laghu-tūla-samāpatteś cākāśa-gamanam

By making *Samyama* on the relation between the *Ākāsa* and the body the Yogi becoming light as cotton wool goes through the skies.

This *Ākāsa* is the material of this body; it is only *Ākāsa* in a certain form that has become the body. If the *Yogi* makes *Samyama* on this *Ākāsa* material of his body, it acquires the lightness of *Ākāsa*, and can go anywhere through the air.

44

बहिरकल्पिता वृत्तिर्महाविदेहा ततः प्रकाशावरणक्षयः

bahir-akalpitā vṛttir-mahā-videhā tataḥ prakāśāvaraṇa-kṣayaḥ

> By making *Samyama* on the real modifications of the mind, which are outside, called great disembodiness, comes disappearance of the covering to light.

The mind in its foolishness thinks that it is working in this body. Why should I be bound by one system of nerves, and put the Ego only in one body, if the mind is omnipresent?

There is no reason why I should. The *Yogi* wants to feel the Ego wherever he likes. When he has succeeded in that all covering to light goes away, and all darkness and ignorance vanish. Everything appear to him to be full of knowledge.

45

स्थूलस्वरूपसूक्ष्मान्वयार्थवत्त्वसंयमाद् भूतजयः

sthūla-svarūpa-sūkṣmānvayārthavattva-saṃyamāt bhūta-jayaḥ

> By making *Samyama* on the elements, beginning with the gross, and ending with the superfine, comes mastery of the elements.

The *Yogi* make *Samyama* on the elements, first on the gross, and then on the finer states. This *Samyama* is taken up more by a sect of the Buddhists. They take a lump of clay, and make *Samyama* on that, and gradually they begin to see the fine materials of which it is composed, and when they have known all the fine materials in it, they get power over that element. So with all the elements, the *Yogi* can conquer them all.

46

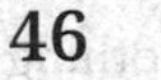

ततोऽणिमादिप्रादुर्भावः कायसंपत्तद्धर्मानभिघातश् च

tato'ṇimādi-prādur-bhāvaḥ kāya-saṃpat-tad-dharānabhighātś ca

> From that comes minuteness, and the rest of the powers, "glorification of the body," and indestructibleness of the bodily qualities.

This means that the *Yogi* has attained the eight powers. He can make himself as light as a particle, he can make himself huge, as heavy as the earth, or as light as the air; he will rule everything he wants, he will conquer everything he wants, a lion will sit at his feet like a lamb, and all his desires be fulfilled at will.

47

रूपलावण्यबलवज्रसंहननत्वानि कायसम्पत्

rūpa-lāvaṇya-bala-vajra-saṃhananatvāni kāya-sampat

The glorifications of the body are beauty, complexion, strength, adamantine hardness.

The body becomes indestructible; fire cannot injure it. Nothing can injure it. Nothing can destroy it until the *Yogi* wishes. "Breaking the rod of time he lives in this universe with his body." In the *Vedas* it is written that for that man there is no more disease, death or pain.

48

ग्रहणस्वरूपास्मितान्वयार्थवत्त्वसंयमादिन्द्रियजयः

grahaṇa-svarūpāsmitāvayārthavattva-saṃyamād-indriya-jayaḥ

By making *Samyama* on the objectivity, knowledge and egoism of the organs, by gradation comes the conquest of the organs.

In perception of external objects the organs leave their place in the mind and go towards the object; that is followed by knowledge and egoism. When the *Yogi* makes *Samyama* on these by gradation he conquers the organs. Take up anything that you see or feel, a book, for instance, and first concentrate the mind on the thing itself. Then on the knowledge that it is in the form of a book, and then the Ego that sees the book. By that practice all the organs will be conquers.

49

ततो मनोजवित्वम् विकरणभावः प्रधानजयश् च

tato mano-javitvam vikaraṇa-bhāvaḥ pradhāna-jayaś ca

> From that comes glorified mind, power of the organs independently of the body, and conquest of nature.

Just as by the conquest of the elements comes glorified body, so from the conquest of the mind will come glorified mind.

50

सत्त्वपुरुषान्यताख्यातिमात्रस्य सर्वभावाधिष्टातृत्वं
सर्वज्ञातृत्वं च

sattva-puruṣānyatā-khyāti-mātrasya sarva-
bhāvādhiṣṭātṛtvaṃ sarva-jñātṛtvaṃ ca

By making *Samyama* on the *Sattva*, to him who has discriminated between the intellect and the *Purusa* comes omnipresence and omniscience.

When we have conquered nature, and realised the difference between the *Purusa* and nature, that the *Purusa* is indestructible, pure and perfect, when the *Yogi* has realised this, then comes omnipotence and omniscience.

51

तद्वैराग्यादपिदोषबीजक्षये कैवल्यम्

tad-vairāgyād-api-doṣa-bīja-kṣaye kaivalyam

By giving up even these comes the destruction of the very seed of evil; he attains *Kaivalya.*

He attains aloneness, independence. Then that man is free. When he gives up even the ideas of omnipotence and omniscience, there will be entire rejection of enjoyment, of the temptations from celestial beings. When the *Yogi* has seen all these wonderful powers, and rejected them, he reaches the goal. What are all these powers? Simply manifestations. They are no better than dreams. Even omnipotence is a dream. It depends on the mind. So long as there is a mind it can be understood, but the goal is beyond even the mind.

52

स्थान्युपनिमन्त्रणे सङ्गस्मयाकरणं पुनरनिष्टप्रसङ्गात्

sthānyupanimantraṇe saṅga-smayākaraṇaṃ punar-aniṣṭa-prasaṅgāt

The *Yogi* should not feel allured or flattered by the overtures of celestial beings, for fear of evil again.

There are other dangers too; gods and other beings come to tempt the *Yogi*. They do not want anyone to be perfectly free. They are jealous, just as we are, and worse than we sometimes. They are very much afraid of losing their places. Those *Yogis* who do not reach perfection die and become gods; leaving the direct road they go into one of the side streets, and get these powers. Then again they have to be born; but he who is strong enough to withstand these temptations, and go straight to the goal, becomes free.

53

क्षणतत्क्रमयोः संयमाद् विवेकजंज्ञानम्

kṣaṇa-tat-kramayoḥ saṃyamād viveka-jam-jñānam

By making *Samyama* on a particle of time and its multiples comes discrimination.

How are we to avoid all these things, these *Devas*, and heavens, and powers? By discrimination, by knowing good from evil. Therefore a *Samyama* is given by which the power of discrimination can be strengthened. This is by making *Samyama* on a particle of time.

54

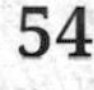

जातिलक्षणदेशैरन्यतानवच्छेदात् तुल्ययोस्ततः प्रतिपत्तिः

jāti-lakṣaṇa-deśair-anyatānavacchedāt tulyayos tataḥ pratipattiḥ

> Those which cannot be differentiated by species, sign and place, even they will be discriminated by the above *Samyama*.

The misery that we suffer comes from ignorance, from non-discrimination between the real and the unreal. We all take the bad for the good, the dream for the reality. Soul is the only reality, and we have forgotten it. Body is an unreal dream, and we think we are all bodies. This non-discrimination is the cause of misery, and it is caused by ignorance. When discrimination comes it brings strength, and then alone can we avoid all these various ideas of body, heavens, and gods and *Devas*. This ignorance arises through differentiating by species, sign or place. For instance, take a cow. The cow is differentiated from the dog, as species. Even with the cows alone how do we make the distinction between one cow and another? By signs. If two objects are exactly similar they can be distinguished if they are in different places. When objects are so mixed up that even these differentiæ will not help us, the power of discrimination acquired by the above-mentioned practice will give us the ability to distinguish them. The highest philosophy of the *Yogi* is based upon this fact, that the *Purusa* is pure and perfect, and is the only "simple" that exists in this universe. The body and mind are compounds, and yet we are ever identifying ourselves with them. That is the great mistake that the distinction has been lost. When this power of discrimination has been attained, man sees that everything in this world, mental and physical, is a compound, and, as such, cannot be the *Purusa.*

55

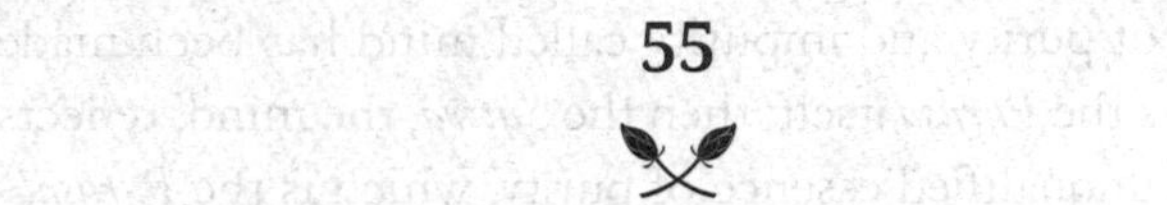

तारकं सर्वविषयं सर्वथाविषयमक्रमं चेति विवेकजं ज्ञानम्

tārakaṃ sarva-viṣayaṃ sarvathā-viṣayam-akramaṃ
ceti vivekajaṃ jñānam

> The saving knowledge is that knowledge of discrimination which covers all objects, all means.

Saving, because the knowledge takes the Yogi across the ocean of birth and death. The whole of Prakriti in all its states, subtle and gross, is within the grasp of this knowledge. There is no succession in perfection by this knowledge: it takes in all things simultaneously, at a glance.

56

सत्त्वपुरुषयोः शुद्धिसाम्ये कैवल्यमिति

sattva-puruṣayoḥ śuddhi-sāmye kaivalyam-iti

By the similarity of purity between the *Sattva* and the *Purusa* comes *Kaivalya*.

When the soul realises that it depends on nothing in the universe, from gods to the lowest atom, that it is called *Kaivalya* (isolation) and perfection. It is attained when this mixture of purity and impurity called mind has been made as pure as the *Purusa* itself; then the *Sattva*, the mind, reflects only the unqualified essence of purity, which is the *Purusa*.

PART IV

KAIVALYA PADA

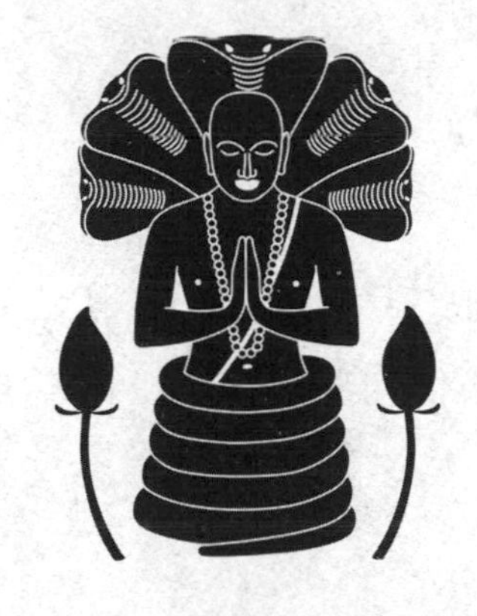

Independence

॥ चतुर्थः कैवल्यपादः ॥

1

जन्मौषधिमन्त्रतपःसमाधिजाः सिद्धयः

janmauṣadhi-mantra-tapaḥ-samādhijāḥ siddhayaḥ

> The *Siddhis* (powers) are attained by birth, chemical means, power of words, mortification or concentration.

Sometimes a man is born with the *Siddhis*, powers, of course from the exercise of powers he had in his previous birth. In this birth he is born, as it were, to enjoy the fruits of them. It is said of *Kapila*, the great father of the *Sānkhya* Philosophy, that he was a born *Siddha*, which means, literally, a man who has attained to success.

The *Yogis* claim that these powers can be gained by chemical means. All of you know that chemistry originally began as alchemy; men went in search of the philosopher's stone, and elixirs of life, and so forth. In India there was a sect called the *Rasāyanas*. Their idea was that ideality, knowledge, spirituality and religion, were all very right, but that the body was the only instrument by which to attain to all these. If the body broke now and then it would take so much more time to attain to the goal. For instance, a man wants to practice *Yoga*, or wants to become spiritual. Before he has advanced very far he dies. Then he takes another body and begins again, then dies, and so on, and in this way much time will be lost in dying and in being born again. If the body could be made strong and perfect, so that it would get rid of birth and death, we should have so much more time to become spiritual. So these *Rasāyanas* say, first make the body very strong, and they claim that this body can be made immortal. The idea is that if the mind is manufacturing the body, and if it be true that each mind is only one particular outlet to that infinite energy, and that there is no limit to each particular outlet getting any amount of power from outside, why is it impossible that we should keep our bodies all the time? We shall have to manufacture all the bodies that we shall ever have. As soon as this body dies we shall have to manufacture another. If we can do that why cannot we do it just here and now, without getting out? The theory is perfectly correct. If it is possible that we live after death, and make other bodies, why is it impossible that we should have the power of making bodies here, without entirely dissolving this body, simply changing it continually? They also thought that in mercury and in sulphur was hidden the most wonderful power, and that by certain preparations of these a man could keep the body as long as he liked. Others believed that certain drugs could bring powers, such as flying through the air, etc. Many of the most wonderful medicines of the present day we owe to the *Rasayamas*, notably the use of metals in medicine. Certain sects of *Yogis* claim that many of their principal teachers are still living in their old bodies. Patanjali, the great authority on *Yoga*, does not deny this.

The power of words. There are certain sacred words called *Mantras*, which have power, when repeated under proper conditions, to produce these extraordinary powers. We are living in the midst of such a mass of miracles, day and night, that we do not think anything of them. There is no limit to man's power, the power of words and the power of mind.

Mortification. You will find that in every religion mortifications and asceticisms have been practised. In these religious conceptions the Hindus always go to the extremes. You will find men standing with their hands up all their lives, until their hands wither and die. Men sleep standing, day and night, until their feet swell, and, if they live, the legs become so stiff in this position that they can no more bend them, but have to stand all their lives. I oncc saw a man who had raised his hands in this way, and I asked him how it felt when he did it first. He said it was awful torture. It was such torture that he had to go to a river and put himself in water, and that allayed the pain for a little. After a month he did not suffer much. Through such practices powers (*Siddhis*) can be attained.

Concentration. The concentration is *Samādhi*, and that is *Yoga* proper; that is the principle theme of this science, and it is the highest means. The preceding ones are only secondary, and we cannot attain to the highest through them. *Samādhi* is the means through which we can gain anything and everything, mental, moral or spiritual.

2

जात्यन्तरपरिणामः प्रकृत्यापूरात्

jātyantara-pariṇāmaḥ prakṛtyāpūrāt

The change into another species is by the filling in of nature.

Patanjali has advanced the proposition that these powers come by first, sometimes by chemical means, or they may be got by mortification and he has admitted that this body can be kept for any length of time. Now he goes on to state what is the cause of the change of the body into another species, which he says is by the filling in of nature. In the next aphorism he will explain this.

3

निमित्तमप्रयोजकम् प्रकृतीनाम् वरणभेदस्तु ततः क्षेत्रिकवत्

nimittam-aprayojakam prakṛtīnām varaṇa-bhedas-tu
tataḥ kṣetrikavat

> Good deeds, etc., are not the direct causes in the transformation of nature, but they act as breakers of obstacles to the evolutions of nature, as a farmer breaks the obstacles to the course of water, which then runs down by its own nature.

When a farmer is irrigating his field the water is already in the canals, only there are gates which keep the water in. The farmer opens these gates, and the water flows in by itself, by the law of gravitation. So, all human progress and power are already in everything; this perfection is every man's nature, only it is barred in and prevented from taking its proper course. If anyone can take the bar off in rushes nature. Then the man attains the powers which are his already. Those we called wicked become saints, as soon as the bar is broken and nature rushes in. It is nature that is driving us towards perfection, and eventually she will bring everyone there. All these practices and struggles to become religious are only negative work to take off the bars, and open the doors to that perfection which is our birthright, our nature.

Today the evolution theories of the *Yogis* will be better understood in the light of modern research. And yet the theory of the *Yogis* is a better explanation. The two causes of evolution advanced by the moderns, *viz.*, sexual selection and survival of the fittest, are inadequate. Suppose human knowledge to have advanced too much as to eliminate competition, both from the function of acquiring physical sustenance and of acquiring a mate. Then, according to the moderns, human progress will stop and the race will die. And the result of this theory is to furnish every oppressor with an argument to calm the qualms of conscience, and men are not lacking, who, posing as philosophers, want to kill out all wicked and incompetent persons (they are, of course, the only judges of competency), and thus preserve the human race! But the great ancient evolutionist, Patanjali, declares that the true secret of evolution is the manifestation of the perfection which is already in every being; that this perfection has been barred, and the infinite tide behind it is struggling to express itself. These struggles and competitions are but the results of our ignorance, because we do not know the proper way to unlock the gate and let the water in. This infinite tide behind must express itself, and it is the cause of all manifestation, not competition for life, or sex gratification, which are only momentary, unnecessary, extraneous effects, caused by ignorance. Even when all competition has ceased this perfect nature behind will make us go forward until everyone has become perfect.

Therefore there is no reason to believe that competition is necessary to progress. In the animal the man was suppressed, but, as soon as the door was opened, out rushed man. So, in man there is the potential god, kept in by the locks and bars of ignorance. When knowledge breaks these bars the god becomes manifest.

4

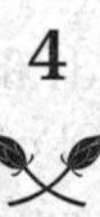

निर्माणचित्तान्यस्मितामात्रात्

nirmāṇa-cittānyasmitā-mātrāt

From egoism alone proceed the created minds.

The theory of *Karma* is that we suffer for our good or bad deeds, and the whole scope of philosophy is to approach the glory of man. All the Scriptures sing the glory of man, of the soul, and then, with the same breath, they preach this *Karma*. A good deed brings such a result, and a bad deed such a result, but, if the soul can be acted upon by a good or a bad deed it amounts to nothing. Bad deeds put a bar to the manifestation of our nature, of the *Purusa*, and good deeds take the obstacles off, and its glory becomes manifest. But the *Purusa* itself is never changed. Whatever you do never destroys your own glory, your own nature, because the soul cannot be acted upon by anything, only a veil is spread before it, hiding its perfection.

With a view to exhausting their Karma quickly, Yogis create Kāya-vyuha, or groups of bodies, in which to work it out. For all these bodies they create minds from egoism.

These are called "created minds", in contradistinction to their original minds.

5

प्रवृत्तिभेदेप्रयोजकं चित्तमेकमनेकेषाम्

pravṛtti-bhede-prayojakaṃ cittam-ekam-anekeṣām

> Though the activities of the different created minds are various, the one original mind is the controller of them all.

These different minds, which will act in these different bodies, are called made-minds, and the bodies made-bodies; that is, manufactured bodies and minds. Matter and mind are like two inexhaustible storehouses. When you have become a *Yogi* you have learned the secret of their control. It was yours all the time, but you had forgotten it. When you become a *Yogi* you recollect it. Then you can do anything with it, manipulate it any way you like. The material out of which that manufactured mind is created is the very same material which is used as the macrocosm. It is not that mind is one thing and matter another, but they are different existences of the same thing. *Asmitā*, egoism, is the material, the fine state of existence out of which these made-minds and made-bodies of the *Yogi* will be manufactured. Therefore, when the *Yogi* has found the secret of these energies of nature he can manufacture any number of bodies, or minds, but they will all be manufactures out of the substance known as egoism.

6

तत्र ध्यानजमनाशयम्

tatra dhyāna-jam-anāśayam

> Among the various *Chittas* that which is attained by *Samādhi* is desireless.

Among all the various minds that we see in various men, only that mind which has attained to *Samādhi*, perfect concentration, is the highest. A man who has attained certain powers through medicines, or through words, or through mortifications, still has desires, but that man who has attained to *Samādhi* through concentration is alone free from all desires.

7

कर्माशुक्लाकृष्णं योगिनस् त्रिविधमितरेषाम्

karmāśuklākṛṣṇaṃ yoginas trividham-itareṣām

> Works are neither black nor white for the *Yogis*; for others they are threefold, black, white, and mixed.

When the *Yogi* has attained to that state of perfection, the actions of that man, and the *Karma* produced by those actions, will not bind him, because he did not desire them. He just works on: he works to do good, and he does good, but does not care for the result, and it will not come to him. But for ordinary men, who have not attained to that highest state, works are of three kind, black (evil actions), white (good actions), and mixed.

8

ततस् तद्विपाकानुगुणानामेवाभिव्यक्तिर्वासनानाम्

tatas tad-vipākānuguṇānām-evābhivyaktir-vāsanānām

> From these threefold works are manifested in each state only those desires (which are) fitting to that state alone. (The others are held in abeyance for the time being.)

Suppose I have made the three kinds of *Karma*, good, bad, and mixed; and suppose I die and become a god in heaven; the desires in a god body are not the same as the desires in a human body. The god body neither eats nor drinks; what becomes of my past unworked *Karmas*, which produce as their effect the desire to eat and drink? Where would these *Karmas* go when I became a god? The answer is that desires can only manifest themselves in proper environments. Only those desires will come out for which the environment is fitted; the rest will remain stored up. In this life we have many godly desires, many human desires, many animal desires. If I take a god body, only the god desires will come up, because for them the environments are suitable. And if

I take an animal body, only the animal desires will come up, and the god desires will wait. What does that show? That by means of environment we can check these desires. Only that *Karma* which is suited to and fitted for the environments will come out. These proves that the power of environment is the great check to control even *Karma* itself.

9

जातिदेशकालव्यवहितानामप्यानन्तर्यं
स्मृतिसंस्कारयोरेकरूपत्वात्

jāti-deśa-kāla vyavahitānām-apyānantaryāṃ smṛti-saṃskārayor-eka-rūpatvāt

> There is consecutiveness in desire, even though separated by species, space and time, there being identification of memory and impressions.

Experiences becoming fine become impressions; impressions revivified become memory. The word memory here includes unconscious co-ordination of past experience, reduced to impressions, with present conscious action. In each body the group of impressions acquired in a similar body only will become the cause of action in that body. The experiences of dissimilar bodies will be held in abeyance. Each body will act as if it were a descendant of a series of bodies of that species only; thus, consecutiveness of desires will not be broken.

10

तासामनादित्वं चाशिषो नित्यत्वात्

tāsām-anāditvaṃ cāśiṣo nityatvāt

Thirst for happiness being eternal, desires are without beginning.

All experience is preceded by desire for becoming happy. There was no beginning of experience, as each fresh experience is built upon the tendency generated by past experience; therefore desire is without beginning.

11

हेतुफलाश्रयालम्बनैः सङ्हीतत्वादेषामभावे तदभावः

hetu-phalāśrayālambanaiḥ saṅgṛhītatvāt-eṣām-abhāve tad-abhāvaḥ

Being held together by cause, effect, support, and objects, in the absence of these is its absence.

These desires are held together by cause and effect; if a desire has been raised it does not die without producing its effect. Then again, the mind-stuff is the great storehouse, the support of all past desires, reduced to *Samskāra* form; until they have worked themselves out they will not die.

Moreover, so long as the senses receive the external objects fresh desires will arise. If it be possible to get rid of these, then alone desires will vanish.

12

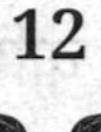

अतीतानागतं स्वरूपतोऽस्त्यध्वभेदाद् धर्माणम्

atītānāgataṃ svarūpato'sti-adhvabhedād dharmāṇām

> The past and future exist in their own nature, qualities having different ways.

The idea is that existence never comes out of non-existence. The past and future, though not existing in a manifested form, yet exist in a fine form.

13

ते व्यक्तसूक्ष्मा गुणात्मानः

te vyaktasūkṣmā guṇātmānaḥ

> They are manifested or fine, being of the nature of the *Gunas.*

The *Gunas* are the three substances, *Sattva*, *Rajas*, and *Tamas*, whose gross state is the sensible universe. Past and future arise from the different modes of manifestation of these *Gunas.*

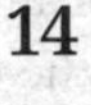

14

परिणामैकत्वाद् वस्तुतत्त्वम्

pariṇāmaikatvāt vastu-tattvam

The unity in things is from the unity in changes. Though there are three substances their changes being co-ordinated all objects have their unity.

15

वस्तुसाम्ये चित्तभेदात् तयोर्विभक्तः पन्थाः

vastu-sāmye citta-bhedāt tayor-vibhaktaḥ panthāḥ

The object being the same, perception and desire vary according to the various minds.

16

तदुपरागापेक्षित्वाच्चित्तस्य वस्तु ज्ञाताज्ञातम्*

tad-uparāgāpekṣitvāc-cittasya vastu jñātājñātam

---

* Swami Vivekananda does not comment on the sutra which is 16th sutra in most versions of *Patanjali's Yoga Sutra.* This sutra is: न चैकचित्ततन्त्रं वस्तु तदाप्रमाणकं तदा किं स्यात् ॥ "An object exists independent of its cognizance by any one consciousness. What happens to it when that consciousness is not there to perceive it?"

Things are known or unknown to the mind, being dependent on the colouring which they give to the mind.

17

सदा ज्ञाताश् चित्तवृत्तयस् तत्प्रभोः पुरुषस्यापरिणामित्वात्

sadā jñātāś citta-vṛttayas tat-prabhoḥ puruṣasyāpariṇāmitvāt

The states of the mind are always known because the lord of the mind is unchangeable.

The whole gist of this theory is that the universe is both mental and material. And both the mental and material worlds are in a continuous state of flux. What is this book? It is a combination of molecules in constant change. One lot is going out, and another coming in; it is a whirlpool, but what makes the unity? What makes it the same book? The changes are rhythmical; in harmonious order they are sending impressions to my mind, and these pieced together make a continuous picture, although the parts are continuously changing. Mind itself is continuously changing. The mind and body are like two layers in the same substance, moving at different rates of speed. Relatively, one being slower and the other quicker, we can distinguish between the two motions. For instance, a train is moving, and another carriage is moving slowly alongside it. It is possible to find the motion of both these, to a certain extent. But still something else is necessary. Motion can only be perceived when there is something else which is not moving. But when two or three things are relatively moving, we first perceive the motion of the faster one, and then that of the slower ones. How is the mind to perceive? It is also in a flux. Therefore another thing is necessary which moves more slowly, then you must get to something in which the motion is still slower, and so on, and you will find no end. Therefore logic compels you to stop somewhere. You must complete the series by knowing something which never changes. Behind this never-ending chain of motion is the *Purusa*, the changeless, the colourless, the pure. All these impressions are merely reflected upon it, as rays of light from a camera are reflected upon a white sheet, painting hundreds of pictures on it, without in any way tarnishing the sheet.

18

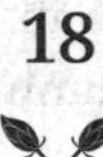

न तत् स्वाभासं दृश्यत्वात्

na tat svābhāsaṃ dṛśyatvāt

Mind is not self-luminous, being an object.

Tremendous power is manifested everywhere in nature, but yet something tells us that it is not self-luminous, not essentially intelligent. The *Purusa* alone is self-luminous, and gives its light to everything. It is its power that is percolating through all matter and force.

19

एकसमये चोभयानवधारणम्

eka-samaye cobhayānavadhāraṇam

> From its being unable to cognise two things at the same time.

If the mind were self-luminous it would be able to cognise everything at the same time, which it cannot. If you pay deep attention to one thing you lose another. If the mind were self-luminous there would be no limit to the impressions it could receive. The *Purusa* can cognise all in one moment; therefore the *Purusa* is self-luminous, and the mind is not.

20

चित्तान्तरदृश्ये बुद्धिबुद्धेरतिप्रसङ्गः स्मृतिसंकरश् च

cittāntara-dṛśye buddhi-buddher-atiprasaṅgaḥ smṛti-saṅkaraś ca

> Another cognising mind being assumed there will be no end to such assumptions and confusion of memory.

Let us suppose that there is another mind which cognises the first, there will have to be something which cognises that, and so there will be no end to it. It will result in confusion of memory, there will be no storehouse of memory.

21

चितेरप्रतिसंक्रमायास् तदाकारापत्तौ स्वबुद्धिसंवेदनम्

citer-apratisaṃkramāyās tad-ākārāpattau svabuddhi-saṃvedanam

The essence of knowledge (the *Purusa*) being unchangeable, when the mind takes its form, it becomes conscious.

Patanjali says this to make it more clear that knowledge is not a quality of the *Purusa*. When the mind comes near the *Purusa* it is reflected, as it were, upon the mind, and the mind, for the time being, becomes knowing and seems as if it were itself the *Purusa*.

22

द्रष्टृदृश्योपरक्तं चित्तं सर्वार्थम्

draṣṭṛ-dṛśyoparaktaṃ cittaṃ sarvārtham

Coloured by the seer and the seen the mind is able to understand everything.

On the one side the external world, the seen, is being reflected, and on the other, the seer is being reflected; thus comes the power of all knowledge to the mind.

23

तदसङ्ख्येयवासनाभिश् चित्रमपि
परार्थं संहत्यकारित्वात्

tad-asaṅkhyeya vāsanābhiś citram-api parārthaṃ saṃhatya-kāritvāt

The mind through its innumerable desires acts for another (the *Purusa*), being combinations.

The mind is a compound of various things, and therefore it cannot work for itself. Everything that is a combination in this world has some object for that combination, some third thing for which this combination is going on. So this combination of the mind is for the *Purusa*.

24

विशेषदर्शिन आत्मभावभावनाविनिवृत्तिः

viśeṣa-darśina ātma-bhāva-bhāvanā-nivṛttiḥ

For the discriminating the perception of the mind as *Atmān* ceases.

Through discrimination the *Yogi* knows that the *Purusa* is not mind.

25

तदा विवेक निम्नं कैवल्यप्राग्भारं चित्तम्

tadā viveka-nimnaṃ kaivalya-prāg-bhāraṃ cittam

Then bent on discriminating the mind attains
the previous state of *Kaivalya* (isolation).

Thus the practice of *Yoga* leads to discriminating power, to clearness of vision. The veil drops from the eyes, and we see things as they are. We find that this nature is a compound, and is showing the panorama for the *Purusa*, who is the witness; that this nature is not the Lord, that the whole of these combinations of nature are simply for the sake of showing these phenomena to the *Purusa*, the enthroned king within. When discrimination comes by long practice fear ceases, and the mind attains isolation.

26

तच्छिद्रेषु प्रत्ययान्तराणि संस्कारेभ्यः

tac-chidreṣu pratyayāntarāṇi saṃskārebhyaḥ

The thoughts that arise as obstructions to that
are from impressions.

All the various ideas that arise making us believe that we require something external to make us happy are obstructions to that perfection. The *Purusa* is happiness and blessedness by its own nature. But that knowledge is covered over by past impressions. These impressions have to work themselves out.

27

हानमेषां क्लेशवदुक्तम्

hānam-eṣāṃ kleśavad-uktam

Their destruction is in the same manner as of ignorance, etc., as said before.

28

प्रसङ्ख्यानेऽप्यकुसीदस्य सर्वथा
विवेकख्यातेर्धर्ममेघसमाधिः

prasaṅkhyāne'pyakusīdasya sarvathā viveka-khyāter dharma-meghas-samādhiḥ

Even when arriving at the right discriminating knowledge of the senses, he who gives up the fruits, unto him comes as the result of perfect discrimination, the *Samādhi* called the cloud of virtue.

When the *Yogi* has attained to this discrimination, all these powers will come that were mentioned in the last chapter, but the true *Yogi* rejects them all. Unto him comes a peculiar knowledge, a particular light called the *Dharma Megha*, the cloud of virtue. All the great prophets of the world whom history has recorded had this. They had found the whole foundation of knowledge within themselves. Truth to them had become real. Peace and calmness, and perfect purity became their own nature, after they had given up all these vanities of powers.

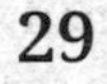

ततः क्लेशकर्मनिवृत्तिः

tataḥ kleśa-karma-nivṛttiḥ

From that comes cessation of pains and works.

When that cloud of virtue has come, then no more is there fear of falling, nothing can drag the *Yogi* down. No more will there be evils for him. No more pains.

तदा सर्वावरणमलापेतस्य ज्ञानस्यानन्त्याज् ज्ञेयमल्पम्

tadā sarvāvaraṇa-malāpetasya jñānasyānantyāt jñeyam-alpam

> Then knowledge, bereft of covering and impurities, becoming infinite, the knowable becomes small.

Knowledge itself is there; its covering is gone. One of the Buddhistic scriptures sums up what is meant by the Buddha (which is the name of a state). It defines it as infinite knowledge, infinite as the sky. Jesus attained to that state and became the Christ. All of you will attain to that state, and knowledge becoming infinite, the knowable becomes small. This whole universe, with all its knowable, becomes as nothing before the *Purusa.* The ordinary man thinks himself very small, because to him the knowable seems to be so infinite.

31

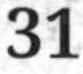

ततःकृतार्थानाम् परिणामक्रमसमाप्तिर्गुणानाम्

tataḥ kṛtārthānaṃ pariṇāma-krama-samāptir-guṇānām

> Then are finished the successive transformations of the qualities, they having attained the end.

Then all these various transformations of the qualities, which change from species to species, cease forever.

32

क्षणप्रतियोगी परिणामापरान्तनिग्राह्यः क्रमः

kṣaṇa-pratiyogī pariṇāmāparānta-nirgrāhyaḥ kramaḥ

> The changes that exist in relation to moments, and which are perceived at the other end (at the end of a series) are succession.

Patanjali here defines the word succession, the changes that exist in relation to moments. While I am thinking, many moments pass, and with each moment there is a change of idea, but we only perceive these changes at the end of a series. So, perception of time is always in the memory. This is called succession, but for the mind that has realised omnipresence all these have finished. Everything has become present for it; the present alone exists, the past and future are lost. This stands controlled, and all knowledge is there in one second. Everything is known like a flash.

33

पुरुषार्थशून्यानां गुणानां प्रतिप्रसवः
कैवल्यं स्वरूपप्रतिष्ठ वा चितिशक्तिरेति

puruṣārtha-śūnyānāṃ guṇānāṃ-pratiprasavaḥ kaivalyaṃ svarūpa-pratiṣṭhā vā citiśaktiriti

> The resolution in the inverse order of the qualities, bereft of any motive of action for the *Purusa*, is *Kaivalya*, or it is the establishment of the power of knowledge in its own nature.

Nature's task is done, this unselfish task which our sweet nurse, Nature, had imposed upon herself. As it were, she gently took the self-forgetting soul by the hand, and showed him all the experiences in the universe, all manifestations, bringing him higher and higher through various bodies, till his glory came back, and he remembered his own nature. Then the kind mother went back the way she came, for others who have also lost their way in the trackless desert of life. And thus she is working, without beginning and without end. And thus through pleasure and pain, through good and evil, the infinite river of souls is flowing into the ocean of perfection, of self-realisation.

Glory unto those who have realised their own nature! May their blessings be on us all!

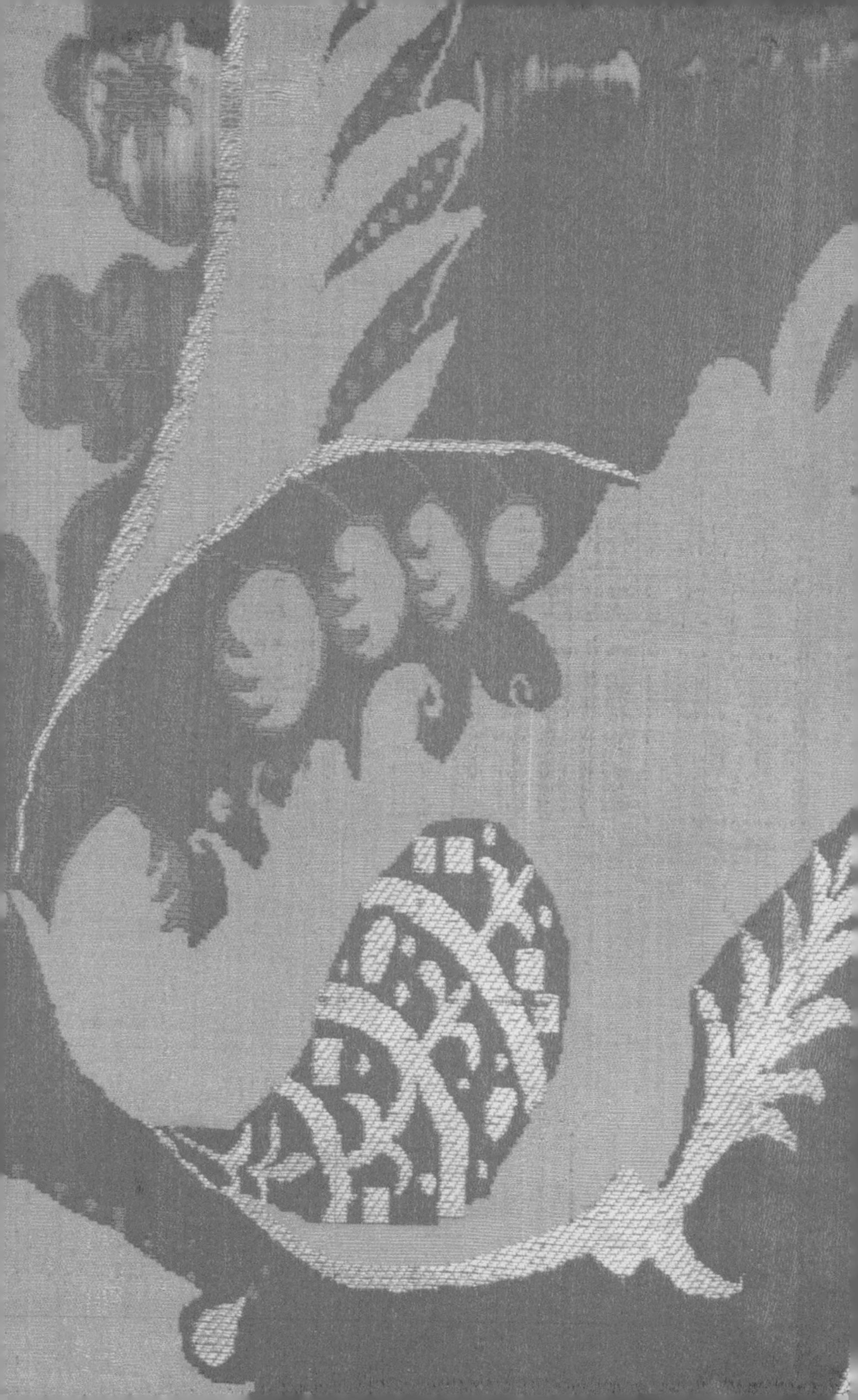